Praise for *8: Rediscovering Life After a Brain Tumor*

In her new book, 8: Rediscovering Life after a Brain Tumor, Nathalie Jacob vividly takes readers on a touching, often unexpectedly humorous, and inspiring journey down the hospital halls and into her new life and "world of 8s," after hearing the shocking words that often make time stand still: "You have a brain tumor." This book will surprise you, delight you, and offer a new perspective on what life throws your way; a must-read for anyone facing what is a seemingly insurmountable challenge.

- **Kimberly Roy-Canning**
  Executive Director, Connecticut Brain Tumor Alliance, Inc.

Nathalie is not only a brain tumor survivor but has managed to re-create her life around a malady called Gerstmann Syndrome. Despite experiencing the major changes in her cognitive abilities, and therefore her life, that the syndrome causes she has managed to tell her story in this book. Her story is a magical weave of tremendous strength along with warm tenderness. It is a wonderful stepping stone for anyone having a similar experience along with being an inspiring story for any of us.

- **Andrea Laudano**
  MSN, APRN. Connecticut, USA.

An extraordinary book by an extraordinary person who has experienced more in 30 years of life than most will in a life-time. A story of triumph over adversities with lessons for all of us to appreciate and embrace our lives. I strongly urge you to read it.

- **Sally Averill IE MBA. London, UK.**

This is a gripping story of somebody that had everything in life and it changed in a matter of days. Nathalie tells this story in an entertaining way. For all of us who are healthy it is just a heads up reminding us that not everything comes out as planned but for those that are enduring these illnesses such courageous experiences can help a lot.

- **Alvaro Sanchez. Bogota, Colombia.**
  Verified Purchase Amazon Review

Great book! I couldn't stop reading it, so I finished it the same day I downloaded it in my Kindle. A real emotional rollercoaster. It was like being on a side with Nathalie the whole time. Thanks for sharing this life changing experience and helping us understand better people with this kind of health issues. Many of us are waiting for second and third part of this story. Please read this book , it is full of love and it is based on an inspiring story.

- **Ricardo Pedraza. MBA IE Business School. Monterey, MEXICO. Verified Purchase Amazon Review**

Inspiring and great read for everyone. I enjoyed the way the author shared so much of herself honestly and objectively. Getting to know her and following along with her journey kept my attention - I read the book in less than 3 days. It has something relatable for everyone - I can't recommend enough. It has inspired me to have more strength and courage and appreciate the little things every day.

- **Kim Roberts. San Francisco, USA.**
  Verified Purchase Amazon Review

A heartfelt story of a woman's struggle through a life changing repercussion to a surgery that took away some of the most important things that identified her. Frustration, patience, love and optimism colors the otherwise grim story within, but well worth the read.

- **Sean Yelle. NYC, USA.**
  Verified Purchase Amazon Review.

Wonderful book! I've read many after my craniotomy, but this one grabs you at the core. I have grown. A Magna Cumme Luade grad, member of Phi Kappa Phi and Beta Gamma Sigma, my education was what I identified with. This book helped me mourn that loss. My cognitive deficits are the new me. She tried so hard and did everything to get that back. Sometimes it is gone, like losing a loved one. Thank you, Nathalie for showing the real trials of going from a vivacious young lady to one with a disability. Reality with more than a dose of hope - emotional healing. I highly, highly recommend.

- **Gordon Pederson. USA.**
  Verified Purchase Amazon Review.

8

Rediscovering Life After a Brain Tumor

NATHALIE JACOB

Visit www.EightMyMemoir.com for more information, pictures and blog conversations with the author.

Authored with Simon Gilbert.

Book cover designed and donated by Anthony Wakeford-Brown. www.magicboxmedia.com

Back cover picture taken by Christian Salvati.

Also available as a eBook.

ISBN-10:1546661832
ISBN-13: 978-1546661832
Library of Congress Control Number: 2017911310
CreateSpace Independent Publishing Platform, North Charleston, SC

To my daughter, my loving husband and my supportive parents; from the bottom of my heart, thank you for loving me, laughing with me and crying with me.

For brain-tumor patients, survivors and caregivers, I hope my journey can make your journey better.

CONTENTS

FORWARD
PREFACE
ACKNOWLEDGEMENTS

FORWARD

I met Nathalie in the summer of 2011 via a conference call. She was interviewing me for a new position in the company where we worked, that had become available in Puerto Rico. I was living in Chiswick, London at the time. I was offered the job, but before accepting I travelled to San Juan to get a feel for the Island, culture and role.

Nathalie kindly gave up her weekend to show me around. I accepted the job, and the rest is history... what I learnt a couple of years later before Nathalie and I were to be married was that when I left the island that day, she had called the general manager to say we should not offer me the job, as I was too boring. It was too late, the offer had been extended and I had accepted, little was she to know that two years later I would propose and she would say yes.

I am immensely proud of Nathalie for writing this memoir. To open yourself up publicly about your life with the purpose to help others is very courageous.

Nathalie has always been courageous. Ever since I met her, she has always been a driven person and has a genuine heart to help those around her. I don't think she discovered her true purpose in life and the strength she had in the latter until after the surgery though. Going on this journey with her, I learnt so much more about her kind heart, high intellect and drive to keep going even when she was at her lowest point. She picked herself up and pushed forwards with belief and perseverance.

Since becoming a mother to our little Nicole, she has blossomed, and whilst the brain tumor side effects are still in our life and will be forever more, she has created a new life, new reality and made the best of it.

This story gives some insight of her journey, and not only helped Nathalie with her therapy but to process the trauma. I hope you enjoy reading it as much as I did.

Simon

PREFACE

I started my journey writing this book in 2016, in Connecticut as a part of my therapy, and finished in the fall of 2018.

I had never intended to publish this book, my vision was to write a memoir of my experience following my brain tumor for my daughter Nicole, so that one day she might understand a bit more about what mommy had gone through, and my life before surgery.

I decided to publish to share my journey with others so I might in some way be able to help them on their journey.

I do not proclaim to be an author, and English is not my first language. Following my surgery I suffered several side effects that effected my cognitive functioning, so there may be some mistakes as you read.

A percentage of the earnings from each sale will go to Brain Tumor Research.

I hope you enjoy.

ACKNOWLEDGMENTS

To my loving husband, no words can describe how thankful I am to you. You have been there for me unconditionally for everything and in every single moment of this journey. You proposed to a woman and ended up with a very different one, yet your love and care for me has never changed. I love you and will for the rest of my life.

To my parents—you kind of expect parents to be there in difficult moments, but I would have never imagined how important it was for me for this to be true. Thank you so much for understanding me, helping me, bathing me and helping me learn to write again. Thank you for still being here for me.

To my family and my husband's family, thank you for being there for me.

A special thank-you to Tasos and Nani for being such good friends before, during, and after the surgery—Tasos for making fun of me on my math abilities and Nani for babysitting me.

My close friends abroad, thank you for supporting me over the phone and making me feel at home, when I was so far from it.

I would like to express my gratitude for my friends and colleagues from Millicom and Diageo for surprising me by being so supportive and generous with me and also with my husband. Thank you!

CHAPTER ONE

8

The nurse and I walked the corridors of Jackson Memorial Hospital and stopped at a door.

"What does the number say?" she asked.

"Eight," I answered.

Continuing to the next door, she asked me. "What number does this door say?"

Without hesitation, "Eight," I answered again. We walked further until I was too tired to go on. "Eight," I answered again.

It was with a journey of eights that I experienced my first walk after my craniotomy.

The day after a two-hour brain surgery, my brain read all numbers as eights. They were *not* eights, but how amazing the brain can be! Since then, I've found it interesting to learn the different meanings of this number, whether it is defined by science, astronomy, or religion. According to a Bible-study website, "The number eight in the Bible represents a new beginning, meaning a new order or creation, and man's true 'born again' event when he is resurrected from the dead into eternal life."[1] Although I'm not a very spiritual person, this one definitely spoke to me.

***

Back in my hospital room, which we nicknamed "the Chateau de Versailles," my husband, dad, and stepmom Antonella helped me back to bed. What a room! I was so lucky. It was enormous and filled with natural light, but I couldn't really enjoy it. I was so sensitive to light after the surgery that we had to keep all the curtains closed. When the doctors came in and asked me to read or write, we had to use a little flashlight.

When I tried to speak, my voice came out like a little girl's—a tiny, squeaky voice. The doctor explained that it was because of a tube used during surgery and it would take a couple of days for my normal voice to return.

My pain was escalating, so they gave me more morphine. Morphine! What a miraculous drug. It's the strangest drug to explain. I don't understand why it was so enjoyable, but when they opened the valve to send some into my veins, I felt a tingling in my arm, and then I slowly fell asleep like a baby. That was it. No pain, only sleep. I don't remember any dreams, hallucinations, or strange side effects, only the feeling that I was sleeping on a bed of clouds, dreaming of sleeping.

Speaking of pain, when the nurses asked me to rate my pain from one to ten, on a scale, guess what number I always answered? "Eight." They showed me a board with smiley faces and pain faces so that I could point at where my pain level was. It seemed that eight was the only number in my visual vocabulary as well.

Back in the hospital room with my father and stepmother, it was time for my first breakfast in forty-eight hours. Oh, how nice

---

[1] The Meaning of Numbers. (2016). Retrieved from
http://www.biblestudy.org/bibleref/meaning-of-numbers-in-bible/8.html.

the eggs tasted! Hospital eggs tasted like any great brunch at a five-star hotel. My brain definitely had me confused but in a good way in this instance.

I had already been in the hospital for two nights and was trying to figure out how much longer my stay would be. I couldn't count. Antonella and my dad patiently helped me do the analysis. I still had four more days in the hospital, though I quickly forgot the answer.

Shortly after breakfast, Dr. Smith arrived to check on me. His Moroccan accent was like music to my ears and his voice filled me with peace and harmony. I don't know whether it was the way he spoke, the fact that I trusted him after he performed a successful surgery on me, or his kind demeanor that comforted me. Probably a mixture of the three, but his compassion since our first meeting was reassuring. A warm heart is so important to a patient in this situation.

He started out with some basic questions, "What year were you born?"

"1830."

"What year is this?"

"Nineteen…something."

"What month is it?"

"No idea."

"Where are you?"

"The hospital."

"Who are these people?"

"My dad and Antonella."

"Who is the president of the United States?"

"Obama."

"Count from one to ten."

"One, two…mmm…three…ten."

"How much is two plus three?"

"Four."

"How much is three plus seven?"

"Wow. That is very difficult."

"Write your name on this paper." He handed me a pen and a white sheet of paper.

I drew a circle over and over and over again and laughed out loud for no reason. That was how I spelled my name for the first time after the surgery.

"Read this sentence for me."

"Mmm…nope. Don't know what it says."

Day two after my surgery. I could not read, write, add, tell right from left (though I have always struggled with this for some reason), or remember when I was born. I guess the usual reaction is worry, sadness, or stress in a situation like this, but not for me. To the amazement of the doctors who crowded around my bed, I couldn't stop laughing and enjoying the moment. I found it fascinating! How can a thirty-four-year-old with an MBA not be able to write her own name? Hilarious!

Dr. Smith explained that I was suffering from "Gerstmann syndrome." The National Institute of Neurological Disorders and Stroke describes it as follows:

Gerstmann syndrome is a type of cognitive

impairment that results from damage to a specific area of the brain—the left parietal lobe in the region of the angular gyrus. It can occur after a stroke or in association with damage to the parietal lobe. It is characterized by four primary symptoms: a writing disability (agraphia or dysgraphia), a lack of understanding of the rules for calculation or arithmetic (acalculia or dyscalculia), an inability to distinguish right from left, and an inability to identify fingers (finger agnosia).

In addition to exhibiting the above symptoms, many adults also experience aphasia (difficulty in expressing oneself when speaking, in understanding speech, or in reading and writing).

There is no cure for Gerstmann syndrome. Treatment is symptomatic and supportive. Occupational and speech therapies may help diminish the dysgraphia and apraxia. In addition, calculators and word processors may help school children cope with the symptoms of the disorder. In adults, many of the symptoms diminish over time.[2]

Dr. Smith noted that my side effects after the surgery where strong. On a scale of zero to ten, with zero representing no side effects and ten representing the worst, I was sitting at an eight. The only Gerstmann syndrome side effect that I didn't have was that I recognized my fingers. Other than that, everything was affected.

Even at this point, I didn't worry at all. With English as my second language, I misinterpreted the word *temporal* for "temporary" and therefore thought that my side effects were

[2] The National Institute of Neurological Disorders and Stroke. (2016). Retrieved from http://www.ninds.nih.gov/disorders/gerstmanns/gerstmanns.htm.

temporary that they wouldn't be there for life. So I decided to enjoy the moment, as I would only be compromised for a period of time and then go back to normal. I decided to enjoy my time "being dumb" while it lasted.

I found the fact that I couldn't read or write intriguing and entertaining. Just some hours before, everything was normal, and now I couldn't read or write. Yet, interestingly enough, I could still speak my three languages, Spanish, English, and French, perfectly.

The only frustrating part of my side effects were the speech impediments. Knowing what I wanted to say but not finding the words to say it was frustrating. Thinking of a word but having another word come out of my mouth was frustrating. Not being able to communicate was frustrating.

I pointed to the curtains, indicating them to my husband.

"You want me to open them?" he asked.

I continued pointing and implying that I did, so he proceeded. But the curtains were not really curtains; rather, they were beige blinds with frosted glass windows behind them. Drawn or not drawn, there was no view to be seen.

My husband opened the blinds.

"No," I said. "The curtains." I could see the perplexed look on Simon's face.

He cautiously drew them back again.

"The curtains," I said again. I was getting more frustrated now, and he could see that I was struggling.

I was trying to say "pillow." I wanted my pillow adjusted, but I was looking at the curtains, so my brain had gone off on its own. We got there, my pillow was adjusted, and I closed my eyes again, as this minor frustration had tired me. I got there with Simon's help.

With the exception of feeling weak from taking medication, I was fine physically, and my ability to move was unaffected.

Dr. Smith had checked my eyesight after the surgery. I couldn't see on the right side, and my peripheral vision for both eyes was gone. He expected my normal vision to return in a month, so I didn't worry about it at this point, thinking, "If it comes back, I can wait as long as it needs." In the meantime, the child's game of peekaboo was a great amusement, as Antonella jumped in and out of my blind spot. It was quite strange that I couldn't see anything to the right, just blackness.

By the time the doctor was leaving my room, my husband arrived. I was so happy to see him. The love of my life, who had been sleeping in an uncomfortable chair beside me for all these days, arrived with exhausted eyes. At least he had been able to run home and shower and get in a short nap before coming back to be with me.

My dad and Antonella shared with Simon the results of Dr. Smith visit—a visit that had been full of laughter, intrigue, and joy for me but was tough for them. It had been difficult for them to see that I was unable to read, write, and spell my name. It had also been difficult to witness that I could no longer remember when I was born or the nickname "Monkey" that I had been calling my husband for years. Of all the many feelings that someone could have had in that moment, I only had two—love for my family and the urge to laugh. My family was feeling just two things as well, but we only shared one in common—love. They were also in total shock.

I was so happy to have my loved ones near me. Being surrounded by the people I loved was definitely the one and only medicine that cured me. I felt so loved and so blessed. How could I not be happy when everything was going so well? After all, I had a successful surgery, was surrounded by my loved ones, and was being taken care of by wonderful doctors and nurses.

The days in the hospital passed quickly. After five days I was ready to be released. I was looking forward to going home. As soon as I stepped outside, I had to wear sunglasses until I was home, as the sun was far too bright for my eyes. On top of that, the noise from the cars and the street was so loud that it seemed as if everything was being amplified through a megaphone. Some people in Miami like to honk their car horns; this pisses me off at the best of times, but now it made me want to cry.

I didn't see the scar from my surgery until two weeks later. It was located on the back side of my head, so unless I stood in front of a mirror and held another mirror behind me, I couldn't see it. I think this was helpful, as I didn't realize what a big scar I had. My ignorance of the matter made me take things more lightly.

CHAPTER TWO

THE COINCIDENTAL FINDING

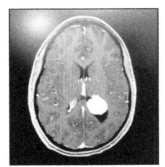

NATHALIE JACOB'S BRAIN MRI, 2015

Two weeks before the surgery, I was heading for my first appointment with Dr. Smith. On the way, I was calm and relaxed, though I could tell Simon was tense. I have always been healthy and have never broken any bones or been sick with anything. I have no allergies and take no medications at all. I was sure that if I had anything, it wasn't anything serious as I had no symptoms. I was as normal as I have always been.

I filled out the papers and waited. When it was finally our turn, Dr. Smith asked me why I was there with a kind look and a fascinating accent.

"Three weeks ago, I went skiing at Whistler with some colleagues."

I love skiing. It's one of my passions in life. On the first day, nothing hurt, and my energy was up and running. I skied like I sometimes do, a bit kamikaze. It hadn't snowed in a while; therefore, the slopes were icy. In the United States, it's common to use helmets, but in Europe it wasn't. I skied the European way, with no helmet. My husband did not approve.

I went down the run, full-on House music with my favorite song on repeat. Next thing I knew, I was tumbling down the hill and ended up hitting my head against the ice. Wow, did it hurt!

I didn't stand up for a couple of minutes. My friends came up to ask me how I was. I had cracked my glasses, and it proved to be lucky because they protected me from hitting my head straight against the ice.

I stood up again and went on skiing. After the fall, I must admit that I was skiing nervously, with a lot of pain in the middle finger of my right hand, but I wasn't about to let a fall to ruin my next few days of skiing. It was only the first day!

I skied significantly slower, because off the fall. If you don't get back on the horse immediately, you never will, I forced myself to ski.

That night, we went to the second-best part of skiing, après-ski! My finger was completely black, but I could move it, so I wrapped it up with tape and continued skiing the rest of the holidays.

Back in Miami, I went back to work for a weak before my next ski trip to Aspen with my husband. As my finger was still black, I didn't want to risk my next trip, so we went to the urgent care next to our house in Coral Gables.

I shared how I had fallen, and they asked me if I had lost consciousness or experienced any nausea or sickness after my fall. I said, "No". They said I looked fine. They x-rayed my finger, and it wasn't broken, only badly bruised. So great! I was up and running, ready for my next ski trip to my favorite place with my favorite person, my husband.

I came down with the flu just after the visit to urgent care. It was the real one that knocks you down for three or four days. Such a simple disease, but the power it has to make you feel really bad is unbelievable! So there I was, counting down the days until the flu was finished.

I was leaving for my ski trip that Friday, but even though the flu had disappeared on Wednesday, I still had an intense headache. I wasn't sure it was still my sinuses, or maybe the ski fall in Whistler. Either way, I didn't want to risk it and went back to the same urgent care just in case.

I explained that I had been there only a week before, and they had found nothing, but I still had headaches after the flu. They checked my sinuses, which were still blocked, and said it was probably that, but they ordered a CAT scan just in case, so I was alone, as Simon was working. I planned to go back to work after the visit, as it was a quick check-up.

The results came about thirty minutes later. "Nothing happened with the ski fall. Nothing at all."

I felt an instant sense of relief, but they hadn't finished yet.

"We found what is called a coincidental finding. You have a mass in the left side of your brain that needs to be checked immediately. Go from here to the nearest hospital if you can drive. If not, we'll call an ambulance. "

What could be that urgent to make me go immediately? I called Simon and told him to meet me at the nearest hospital as soon as he could. "Do not pass go; do not collect two hundred dollars," as he would say.

Once in the hospital I was asked to put on a hospital gown and was passed from one doctor to another for four hours. I repeated the same story to each of them, finally getting the doctor to tell me, "This is not an emergency. We don't treat you here. You need to book an appointment with a neurologist."

Oh well, the system definitely seems to work in an impractical, disorderly way sometimes.

So I went back to work to finish off my last day before going to Aspen the following morning. In the meantime, I booked my first appointment with Dr. Smith for as soon as I was back from Aspen.

***

At the doctor's office with Simon, I told Dr. Smith the complete story and that I was sure I had nothing and that it was something harmless.

Dr. Smith said, "You have a benign brain tumor, an intraventricular meningioma of three to four centimeters." He showed me the MRI results on the computer screen.

This still didn't mean anything to my husband or me.

"My recommendation is to operate as soon as possible. If the meningioma is not removed, it will continue growing, and, even though there have been no side effects yet, it is just a matter of time until you will have them. There is about a twenty percent risk with the surgery temporarily affecting the peripheral view on the right side. It's only permanent two percent of the time."

At that moment, Simon and I did get a bit concerned. Surgery. Wow. But I was perfect! It is such a controversial feeling to think of having to have a brain surgery to "fix me"—but fix me from what? I was perfect! Simon and I grabbed hands, and our eyes got watery—not because we were worried, but because we didn't expect this. Especially not me, with my "everything is perfect" attitude.

Dr. Smith was kind and let us breathe a bit before we had more questions. But we were so startled that barely any questions came into our heads besides basic ones, like when I would be able to go back to work. He said I could go back in three weeks, which made me think it was a piece of cake then. It must be a straightforward surgery with barely any recovery time.

Regarding the peripheral view with only a 2 percent chance for it to be serious, what were the odds that it would be a side effect for me? Close to none! So no worries at all on this matter.

Cool! I was back to the positive. It was definitely a short surgery and an easy, short recovery.

Dr. Smith told us his head nurse would contact us later that day with more instructions prior to the surgery. He also mentioned a private room was not guaranteed, but he would try his best to have one for me.

As we exited through the waiting room, we passed a lady with what must have been a ten-inch scar on her head, seemingly from a recent brain surgery. I didn't even consider this would be how mine would look. It hadn't even crossed my mind—and still didn't.

This was the first visit with him and the last before going into surgery.

We left Dr. Smith's office, and, in the car, we called my dad and Antonella and told them how the visit went. Simon and I were calm, but my dad and Antonella were nervous. I was telling them in a jokey way, but they were quite serious about it. I guess that, unlike me, they understood the significance of this, while I, a bit naïve, didn't.

As soon as I told them, they immediately booked flights to come and be with us. This was in less than two weeks' time! After I spoke to them, I also called my mom to tell her. She also wanted to come and be with me, but my parents didn't get along. They simply despised each other. Having them in the same place at the same time would stress me more than help me. So I preferred to have them come and support me, but not at the same time.

We drove back to the office building together because even though Simon and I worked for different companies, they were on different floors of the same building.

I felt so bad that I had to ask permission to take a sick leave. I had only been working for Millicom for six months, but they were great. My boss, Adam, is a genuine and kind human being. I knew that my not being there would mean more work for him and Teddy, my colleague, who is also an incredible person.

As soon as I arrived in the office, Adam asked me how the visit went with the doctor. I shared with him, and he was very positive like me. He said everything would be OK, and, of course I could take the time off I needed to recover. (I told him it would be three weeks, as the doctor said.) He recommended that I go to speak to human resources, as Millicom had just implemented a short-term leave program with the insurance company, and I probably needed to fill out some paperwork.

Handing in my role for three weeks…

Maybe an hour or two later, Linda (Dr. Smith's head nurse) called me to go over the details of what I needed to bring to the hospital: comfortable pajamas and underwear. They also told me that I couldn't take any aspirin until the surgery (it acts as a blood thinner), I couldn't drink any alcohol for seventy-two hours before or eat any food for six hours before. She mentioned something different from what Dr. Smith had said in terms of how long I would be away from work. She said that Dr. Smith was always very positive, but I needed to ask for five weeks of sick leave, not three.

Right after she told me, I was a bit shaken. But oh well, more time to rest. Not bad! When I told Adam, he said to take all the time I needed.

At the end of the day, I knew I had three basic priorities for the next two weeks before the surgery:

1. Accelerate all the pending work I could finish in two weeks and plan a correct and proper handover for the five weeks I would be gone.
2. Buy comfortable hospital pajamas and Crocs to walk around.
3. Buy food so that when my dad and Antonella arrived while I was in the hospital, they would find everything they needed for them and Simon.

As for Simon, he also had some priorities. We needed to change the air conditioning in time for the surgery, and we were in the process of building a swimming pool, so we had to accelerate the process so that the loud, heavy banging would be finished before the surgery. There were so many things for both of us to do in these two weeks.

You will notice that researching the surgery and aftercare was not part of our agenda. It didn't occur to us to research the surgery or after care.

CHAPTER THREE

NATHALIE
MISSPELLED

I was working so frantically that the two weeks flew by. My dad and Antonella arrived on Thursday, March 7, and the fun family time began! The last days of drinking, eating, and being happy to be together. Our all-time favorite restaurant in Miami is Houston's (Hillstone, but we still call it by its old name). So we went twice in those two days: Once with Simon on the day they arrived, and then again on the last day when I could still drink. Simon stayed home because he got a heavy cold. We were worried that the hospital wouldn't let him in due to his cold, but they did, if he wore a mask.

Sunday, March 8, 5:00 p.m. Time to head to the hospital. After so many days of laughing, drinking, eating, and working, it was finally time to leave the house with my little hospital bag, wearing my sweat pants and pink fluffy Crocs. Simon, with his face mask, looked sicker than I did.

We arrived at the Jackson Memorial Hospital in Miami to find ourselves lost. It was Sunday. There was only one person at the reception desk, the guard. The four of us started to understand that this was actually happening (when we said we came to check in for the night), it was my first time checking in to something besides a hotel or flight.

The guard called the supervisor, who guided us to a nice Bupa reception room, where we started filling out the papers. I put on the little white hospital bracelet. Upon reading the bracelet, we noticed that my name was spelled incorrectly. The supervisor verified my information, but the *H* was missing in my first name: *Natalie* instead of *Nathalie*. We pointed it out to the man at reception and he said he would correct it in the file. We waited for maybe forty minutes and then he accompanied us to my room for the night.

We were guided to my room but it wasn't only *my* room. There was another woman there, as I had a shared room.

Though I had never been in a hospital before, having to share a room and a bathroom was uncomfortable. I can imagine that anyone who has to share a room must feel uneasy. Don't misunderstand me. I feel lucky that I had medical insurance and that I had the opportunity to have great care in a great hospital. It was just a bit uncomfortable to share rooms and bathrooms with someone I didn't know.

I had the bed that faced the window. We closed the curtain that splits the room in two, to give ourselves privacy and we tried to keep our voices down so we wouldn't disturb my roommate. I come from a loud, outgoing family. My dad hears 60 percent less than average, and two of my other sisters and I hear 20 to 30 percent less than average. We all basically scream to each other so that we can hear each other, but also because we don't realize we're talking so loudly.

I think this was the first time I ever saw my dad eat McDonald's. Well, he didn't really eat it. He bought it (as there was nothing else available for dinner in the area), ate one fry, and then left the rest. The meal was strange; we were all hungry but couldn't bring ourselves to eat.

And that's when it hit me. The mixture of sitting in a real hospital bed for the first time in a shared room, knowing I had to eat my last meal quickly before my "meal curfew" made me feel uneasy. I couldn't imagine staying there alone. It terrified me! We asked the nurse if it was possible for Simon to stay with me that night. She checked and they allowed him. My roommate was also OK with it, which I was so grateful for!

Many nurses came during the next couple of hours. They checked my blood pressure, took some samples, and explained that we would have to do an MRI (magnetic resonance imaging) later that night when the machine would be available. Every nurse checked if my personal information was correct every time. We told them that my name was misspelled. It was missing an *H*.

We asked if we would see Dr. Smith, but they said we would see him tomorrow morning. I would be the first surgery of the day at 7am. They would come to pick me up at 5:30am. The anesthesiologist came to ask more questions and a doctor came to put some strange circular stickers that looked like Polo candies on the left side of my head.

I realized that all of this was actually happening. I was actually going to have brain surgery in a few hours. We were quite lighthearted in the room. We introduced my dad to his new B&O headphones and joked about going for more steak and champagne.

I was very nervous, until Simon suddenly popped a joke that made us all laugh so much that we completely relaxed again and forgot about the surgery. Simon took a picture of me to show me how I looked with the foam circle stickers on my head and compared it to a mint Polo ad. They were identical! The same side exactly. So time passed by and it was time for them to leave. We kissed good-bye and that would be the last time I'd see them until after the surgery.

Now it was Simon and I, and my roommate. I changed into the hospital gown they gave me, gave all my personal belongings to Simon, and he put them in my bag. He cuddled with me in the hospital bed all night—except when we got interrupted at one in the morning to go for my long-awaited MRI. When the nurses came to pick me up, they pushed me in the same hospital bed. It was the first hospital-bed ride of my life. It was quite amazing to be pushed on a bed.

I went into the MRI. These machines make horrible noises. My father describes them as being inside a plane in World War II, with the guns shooting full-on. "Traka-traka-traka-traka." They offered music, but I couldn't even hear it as the machine noise was so loud, especially since it was a brain MRI, so my head was in the middle of the machine. I never open my eyes when I go into them. I'm not claustrophobic but just in case, I prefer to keep my eyes closed and ignore being inside a tube for forty-five minutes. In the meantime, at least I was covered in blankets and warm, but poor Simon, sick and with a mask on, was freezing, standing outside waiting for the MRI to finish. The love of my life, my hero, was there waiting for me.

We headed back to the room for a bit more of cuddly sleep in the hospital bed. The nurse came to wake us up at 5:30am sharp. She asked me to wash myself with iodine in sponges. I had to rub this wet, cold liquid everywhere on me. Then I put on a different type of hospital gown and onto a different hospital bed. It was time for that last ride before the surgery. Simon walked with me along the bed all the time. I was so tired and sleepy; I wasn't awake enough to feel nervous at this point.

They checked that my information was correct again. For the third time, we said it was correct, except my name was misspelled. It was missing the *H*. They said they would correct it.

Dr. Smith had arrived! He kindly placed his hand on my shoulder and asked how I was feeling. My dad and Antonella returned at 7:30am, just before I was about to move rooms again.

I was now in the pre-surgery room. Dr. Smith went over the details again with my dad, Antonella, and Simon and said he expected it to be a two- to four-hour surgery. He asked me if everything was OK, and we told him that my name was misspelled (which we had mentioned several times already). Oh boy, was he mad—not at us, but at the staff, and with good reason. They could not operate on me with my name incorrectly spelled. So we had to postpone the surgery until the admin staff corrected the misspelling. It took them about an hour to correct, and this time we were finally ready to head in. This extra time gave me the opportunity to see my dad and Antonella before I was sent to the operating room.

The staff said they were taking me in. At that moment, I kissed my family good-bye and they took me into surgery. I was calm. Not many thoughts went through my mind at that point. I knew I was in good hands. They placed the general-anesthesia mask on me and before I even started to count…I passed out.

CHAPTER FOUR

LIFE BEFORE A BRAIN TUMOR

The day I went into surgery, I was thirty-four years old. I was born in Bogota, Colombia but was raised in an international family. My father is French/Colombian and my mother is American who was born in Puerto Rico. One of the great advantages to this was that I had three nationalities, three passports (American, Colombian, and French/EU) since the day I was born and I have had the freedom to live and work in many countries.

Being raised with different cultures and customs in the house has made me an international person but I also never really felt like I belonged 100 percent to any of the countries. For example, even though I was raised in Colombia for most of my childhood, I don't like most Colombian food, the music like *vallenatos,* or the Colombian Christmas traditions like *novenas*. My mom has a Puerto Rican accent and eats more American style while my dad has a

French accent and eats more French style.

When I lived in Colombia, I didn't feel very Colombian and my friends who knew me don't see me as being very Colombian. But when I lived abroad—for example, in France— my Colombian/Latin personality and traditions pop out more than the other nationalities I have. I love Colombia, but I also love France and the United States. I have always defined myself more in percentages—50 percent Colombian, 25 percent American, and 25 percent French.

My French side arrived in Colombia when my great-grandmother who died in Bogota at 106 years of age, and her husband decided to leave Europe just before World War II began. They had a textile company in Lyon and decided to embark on a journey with their two sons (my grandfather and his younger brother), all their employees and their machines in search of peace and a more stable future. It was 1933.

They spent three months crossing the Atlantic and arrived on the coast of Colombia, where they navigated down the river with the heavy equipment on a long journey to Bogota, the capital. My grandfather was eight years old at the time.

They settled in Colombia and once the war was over, they sent their two children to France to finish high school in a boarding school. The boys regularly came back to Colombia to visit their mother and father.

My grandfather met my grandmother in Colombia. She is 100% French as well. Her father was a French diplomat working in Colombia at the time when they met, when they fell in love and got married. He went to Massachusetts Institute of Technology (MIT) to study and came back to Colombia to continue the family business.

He went on to sell it and create a new business, which is now one of the biggest companies in Colombia. He was a very admirable man, the smartest I've ever known. He also was awarded the Legion d'honneur by the French government.

As a great mathematician and a genius, he was a workaholic and quite cold and demanding of his children and grandchildren. When we were teenagers, he was against us even going to the cinema. His theory was that until we graduated from college, our only priority should be to study and only study.

Behind every great man there is an even greater woman, and this could not be truer than in this case, my grandmother, or, as I call her, *Mamo*. In French, *maman* means *mother*. As I heard my father call her mother, I repeated that. From that moment on, all the granddaughters called her *mamo*. My grandmother is the kindest, most elegant, generous, (red-haired) loving human being on the planet. She is full of energy and always positive. Even when my grandfather died of lung cancer, she remained positive, smiling and strong. She is ninety but looks ten years younger. She drives, walks more than I do, has more energy, and a significantly busier social life than I do. She's even been on Facebook longer than I have. She keeps up with world news, culture, and the Internet. She travels once a year to Paris.

On my other side, my grandfather died when my mom was only a girl and I have seen my grandmother once in my life. From a distance, she has been generous towards me and Simon. My mother is the youngest. Her eldest sister lives in Greece, as she married a Greek man, and has two lovely children who are years younger than me and live in Athens.

Two special people have been my maternal great-grandfather

and great-grandmother, who were loving and caring to their four great grandchildren. I met my great-uncle in Spain for the first time later in life, and, since then, I have a deep admiration and love for him and his wife. He is a war hero from Vietnam. When my mother told me that he was part of a great film about the Vietnam War, I didn't believe her until she showed me a clip from a Puerto Rican newspaper. It explained that Mel Gibson was the lead actor in the movie *We Were Soldiers* and a Puerto Rican war hero was being represented in it. How cool is that? He was on the set with Mel Gibson, explaining how it was in the war in Vietnam so that he could portray it as realistically as he could. Last week, my great-uncle was again on TV on AARP, sharing his experience as part of the first battle of Vietnam, the Battle of la Drang. My great-grandfather was a colonel from West Point and so was Tony, his son, my great-uncle. I had a brave family.

My father was born in Colombia but was raised mostly in France in a boarding school, as my grandfather was. He went to study business administration at Boston University, where he met my Puerto Rican mom, Nita, who was studying literature. She wanted to study law after college, but love swept them away and they got married. They finished their degrees and left for Colombia. So that's how my Puerto Rican and French sides ended up in Colombia. I have three younger sisters: Jessica and Loreana are identical twins who are two years younger than me and Marie, the redhead, who is seven years younger. I am the oldest, but, ironical, I am the smallest, at only five feet.

Until I was sixteen years old, we all had a healthy, happy family life. We lived in the same house in the city during our childhood and on the weekends, we went to our house in the countryside, near a lake where we sailed and water skied. Sailing was a family passion. My grandfather was one of the first to bring the sport to Colombia. With four daughters, my parents, we drove in a Volkswagen Type 2 (minibus). Ah…those great 1990s.

During the week, we were good students and good girls and on the weekends, we were sailing and training for championships. I won my first Colombian National Cup in Optimist when I was eleven years old, and I won it again when I was twelve. I lost first place to my sister Loreana for two years in a row but won it again when I was fifteen. It was tough at the time to lose to my sister, it hits your ego, but in a way I'm happy I did because it taught me to be stronger and get better. At that point, I changed sailboats, as the rule in Optimist allowed you to compete only until fifteen. It was fun to do the same sports together, but when I have children of my own, I'm not sure I will put them in competition against each other. I think competition is important but I'm not sure it's good within the same family.

As you can imagine, we were quite the phenomenal sailing family at the time, as nobody could beat the sisters, regardless of which sister was winning. My father was the strongest sailor of us all and he continues to sail in competition every weekend. I can't even count how many national and international competitions he has been in. He is an admirable sportsman—not only in sailing but also in water and snow skiing, gym, golf, and any sport you put him in. He's a hyperactive man who can't sit and watch a movie without standing up after fifteen minutes. He has always been in better shape than any of his daughters. My dad pushed us into competitions and when we didn't feel like sailing, he threatened to sell our sailboats if we stopped. I'm grateful that he pushed us as this is what made us such good sailors.

Sailing is a great sport, but I always saw it only as a sport, never as a career. I was the nerd of the family, always reading, always studying, and always looking for a better school to be in. I was also the ugly, chubby duck of the family. The twins were superhot and popular cheerleaders who were always surrounded by the cute guys and boyfriends. I never had a boyfriend or even kissed a boy until I was sixteen, as I was "the nerd." I was a more conservative, zero-parties, only-study type of girl.

I must admit that I felt insecure and traumatized by silly things like my weight in my teenage years. I was always on a diet, though I stuffed myself with chocolate at night, when nobody would see me. I had humongous boobs, which you might think was a good trait, but when I was twelve to fourteen years old, boys just made fun of me, so I tried to hide them under big, bulky sweatshirts.

The one good thing about being the ugly, chubby one was that it built my personality. If looks wouldn't make me friends, hopefully my personality would. I had a good childhood, but my better years were definitely later in life. I wish Mark Zuckerberg would have been "out there" when I was in high school with his mind-set of "be the nerd." I completely agree with him and think it's the way we should all educate our children, instead of the superficial and wrong way modern society does with pushing teenagers to be hot and popular, which brings no values to adulthood whatsoever.

In preschool and middle school, I attended a private, high-end, American school in Colombia. I started high school in my twin sisters' school, an all-girls' school, but the education level was average, and I was looking for the best education possible. I changed to what was, at the time, the best school for girls, the Nena Cano, which had delivered the best national ICFES (the Colombian equivalent of the SAT) for thirty years. It was fun to be surrounded by other "nerds." The school was such a study place that there were barely any sports. It was 100% focused on intellectual academics.

When I turned sixteen, I went to live in Paris, in search of an even-better education and also to learn French. My best friend at the time was a classmate at the Nena Cano. Her mom transferred to Paris for work, and my friend started studying at Lycée International de Saint-Germain-en-Laye.[3] I applied too and was accepted. It is located on the outskirts of Paris in a lovely town with a castle in the center of it. I lived with a family for two years, to whom I paid room and board. I dedicated 100% of my time to study. This was really the peak of my "nerdy moment." I learned French in three months and went up to the top of my class during that year.

I also continued sailing a lot on the weekends. I was training to qualify for the Olympics, so I got into a class of sailboat that didn't exist in Colombia called *Europe*, which is an all-girls Olympic class. I was so dedicated and passionate that every weekend I traveled three hours by train, plus one hour by bus, and thirty minutes walking on Friday nights and returned late Sunday night to train for two days in Cherbourg in Normandy, the northeast, coldest part of France. Looking back at the time, I'm amazed at all that effort. I could never do that now. It was a really hard year of training. Traveling for so many hours while studying nonstop was exhausting. I also wasn't used to sailing in such cold and harsh conditions.

Communication was not what it is now, so writing letters was the way to go, but they took forever to arrive in Colombia. I was still learning French, my sailing terminology in French was non-existent and only one of the people who sailed in Cherbourg spoke English, so it was difficult to make friends and communicate. I felt lonely there but never lost sight of my goal.

---

[3] Wikipedia contributors. "Lycée International de Saint-Germain-en-Laye". Wikipedia, The Free Encyclopedia. (2015). https://en.wikipedia.org/wiki/Lycée_International_de_Saint-Germain-en-Laye.

The *Europe*-class boat was difficult as well. My intention was sailing, but most of the time I spent swimming! It was a never-ending tipping experience. It was an unstable boat to control, and, as soon as the wind was a bit high, the boat capsized and I ended up swimming after it and getting in again.

Bruises, colds and tears were part of my sailing routine alone in my boat. I often thought of quitting, but my dad had done so much to set me up to be able to train and bought me a boat there, so I couldn't quit.

Being young definitely gave me a lot of energy and motivation. I could compete in the French national sailing championships due to my French passport, but if I intended to qualify for the Olympics, I would do so for the Colombian team. This never happened though.

During my second year in France, I met Michael, my first boyfriend. We were in the same class, so we studied together all the time. As I had no family in France, our relationship was much more intense than a traditional relationship at seventeen years old…and teenagers are already intense! We were together for a bit less than a year and he proposed to me with a lovely gold ring with a sapphire, as blue was my favorite color. His family had been kind, generous and loving with me from the beginning.

On April 22, 1997, I went for a one-week sailing training trip to the south of France, as I had been sponsored as the captain of a five-person boat. The sponsorship was to sail in the biggest high-school regatta in France, where more than five hundred students participated.

Before the train left, I called Michael from a phone booth to let him know that I loved him, missed him enormously and was looking forward to seeing him. I told him the time my train was arriving, as he had offered to pick me up at the station with his mom, Katy. When I arrived at the station, neither he nor Katy were there. My friends offered to give me a ride, but I knew Michael would arrive, so I told them to leave without me. By one in the morning, I thought it was strange that they hadn't arrived yet, but maybe he had misunderstood the time of my arrival, so I took a cab and went home. I didn't call them. I thought it would be rude to call him at that time.

The next day I went to school expecting to find him in class, but when the last student came in and he was still missing, I thought it was odd. I left class and called his house but no one answered the phone. I started to worry, so I left school, took my blue scooter and drove to his house. There was no one there, so I drove to his grandmother's house in Maisons Lafitte. Only his grandmother was there, looking quite pale.

"Where is Michael?" I asked.
"In the hospital," his grandmother answered.
"In the hospital? But why? Is he OK? Can I go and see him?'
"I prefer if you wait for his parents to arrive. They're on their way."

I waited for them to arrive. After a thirty-minute wait his both parents arrived. They sat down beside me on the living-room sofa, his mother took my hands, looked me directly in the eyes, and said, "Michael is dead."

My mind went blank. Blank except for the one thought I had. *Wait, let me ask him. Let me talk to him.* Shock. I was completely in shock. I couldn't think of anything. I had a freezing-cold feeling through my spine. What? Dead? What did that mean, dead? No! It was clearly impossible. Nope, it wasn't happening. He was a young, healthy, strong, athletic, intelligent man. No, there was no way he could be…no.

Michael had been dead for almost a day, but I first found out on

April 23.

My life as I knew it had ended and the man I was going to marry had died. I didn't see any future. It was like somebody had pulled the rug under me and I had only a big black hole to go into with no hope.

To explain how Michael died, how those next months were, and the effects it had on me and his family, I would need to write another book.

The two months after his death are completely blurry and have almost disappeared from my memory. I just have some snapshots but no details. I don't understand why but maybe the brain eliminates memories when we're in shock. My mom spoke to a psychiatrist who recommended that I should go back to Colombia, as a shock like this would be too difficult to bear alone. I could be at risk of falling into a deep depression. So I went back, continued high school and graduated.

Being back in Colombia was tough. My mind was elsewhere. The utter devastation that I was feeling haunted me for more than a year. A couple of times that I was so sad I fainted, and it took me time to process and get back to a normal sense of reality again. At any age, processing loss is tough and is hard for anyone to understand unless they have been through it themselves. My new group of friends in Bogota helped me a lot. Looking back now, I learnt that this was a pivotal moment in my life that helped to shape me for who I am today.

I still maintain a very special relationship with Michael's family, which I consider my own. I truly love them, feel their pain, and we have a supernatural link of love and trust created by the loving memory of Michael.

When I returned to Colombia from France, my parents were separated. They decided to divorce around the same time that Michael died. Michael's death made the divorce easier on me, as I was dealing with a much bigger tragedy. It was a hateful divorce that affected their lives, their families and especially their daughters in the most selfish way. Parents' egos get in the way and blind them to the effects they have on their children when they take their divorce into such a dark place. They never intentionally wanted to hurt us, but the way they managed their divorce affected their four daughters in different ways.

I arrived at my mother's new, rented apartment in Bogota, where she had started to live with Marie, my youngest sister. The twins were living with my father in the house we lived in before. After a fight with my mom over her house rules, she packed all their clothes in trash bags and sent them to live with my father. The twins never rebuilt a relationship with her, even to this day. When they turned eighteen, they left for Paris, to learn French and go to college. In parallel, my father entered a relationship with Antonella, his present wife, and married her.

Part of what made the divorce so dramatic was the process of legally closing the company that my parents had created more than ten years earlier. They both blamed the other and neither wanted to split it equally. The process of what went to who was a complete mess. They both accused the other of theft, lying, cheating and unfairness.

They spent thousands on lawyers, trying to bring each other down. Unfortunately, they did not keep this to themselves but instead, always put us, the daughters, in the middle of the conversation. They tried to convince us who was right and wrong, who hurt the other one more or less, who was lying and who was not. Putting us in the position of choosing which parent to believe also created a separated set of sisters. In the end, who would you believe? All we had were their conflicting stories, and each story was different.

The twins were 100% with my father and Antonella. When they left for France, Marie got into a fight with my mom and also went to live with my dad and Antonella. The fight was over Marie not obeying my mom's rules in the house, which were what she thought were the correct way of bringing someone up. My mom kicked Marie out hoping she would rethink her behavior, but she didn't come back.

Marie also stopped having a relationship with my mother for years. She finished high school in Colombia and left to study in France when she turned eighteen. As she moved into my father's house when she was around thirteen, she had more of a mother-daughter relationship with Antonella. During that time, she also became 100% on my father's side, and 0% on my mom's side.

This separation of the daughters into "political parties" ended, unfortunately, with me being the only one living with my mom and actually having a relationship with her. I must admit that I didn't quite accept Antonella at the time and it took some years for me to accept her. I tried to not take sides, but even though I didn't, the family did. As I was the only one out of four who was living with my mom, my father's family took it as me being against them. We were either in or out, and by being the only one not in, I was out.

For years, I didn't have a relationship with my dad, Antonella, the twins, or my grandparents. Not a strong relationship at least. I wasn't even invited to my father's wedding with Antonella. This situation lasted approximately four or five years. I remained close to Marie though.

The lawsuits lasted forever. There were even some attempts to involve the daughters in lawsuits against the parents, too. The lawsuit fever finally ended maybe ten years after their divorce. My parents still despise each other and don't speak and they have never tried to make peace. By now, we, the daughters, are used to this. It's our "normal." Two people who were passionately in love and had four daughters now can't stand each other.

The support I had from my mom was great. We built a strong relationship. She was the only person I had in that period of my life. We were great friends as well; we told each other everything. My friends also got along well with her, and so did my boyfriends.

She remarried a nice Colombian man, who was generous and kind to her. She started to get a bit closer with Marie as well.

My new life was going well. I missed my father's family, but at least I had a solid relationship with my mom that gave me strength and support in life. I studied business administration in Colombia at the best college in the country, Universidad de los Andes. The nerd in me diminished during college. Graduation was still a priority, just not in the excessively nerdy way I was in school. I became more social, made friends, and had boyfriends. It was a more normal teenage life. I partied, but I was never too crazy. I kept to the normal drinking parties but didn't do drugs. I did once take my car (the one my mom had given me) without permission and 12 hours to the coast of Colombia, down through the arduous mountain range. That was probably the one time I misbehaved; but still, isn't this normal within the teenage years?

In Colombia, and especially in Bogota (where most colleges are), it is culturally normal for kids to live with their parents until they marry or at least have been working for four or five years after graduation. You never see adults younger than twenty-seven living by themselves. I know in Europe and the United States this is uncommon, and by eighteen, many have left their homes, especially as many go to study to different cities or states. Sharing this context is important to understand what happened next.

When I was 22 years old, I went for a six-month Erasmus program to Maastricht, the Netherlands, a little town full of students. I would come back for my last semester before graduation.

While I was away, my boyfriend that lived in Colombia, wanted to help me have a better relationship with my father and he met with him. I don't know what they spoke about, but it worked! When I came back from Maastricht, my dad was open to having a relationship with me, which we started to rebuild little by little.

My mother lost it. Maybe it was the fear of losing the last child she had to my father. She wouldn't admit this at all; it's just my theory. She kicked me out of the house when she saw that I was rebuilding my relationship with my father and Antonella. Of course, her version is different from mine, but regardless of the version, I was out of the house, I was only earning $250 a month at my internship at Frito-Lay, which was barely enough to live.

I asked her why she wanted me out several times. She said she wanted peace and calm at that moment in life. She said I was a smart woman, and I would be very successful and she wished that in the future I would remember that I had a mother. But from that moment on, I would not anymore. She said I could keep some things she had given me like the pillows, DVD player, mattress, etc, but after a long night with no sleep, she didn't allow me to take anything. So I was out with my clothes and had to build a life myself.

I hadn't told my dad anything until the day I had nowhere to sleep. I didn't want to share this because of the history between them, but I needed to. I didn't have anywhere to go. My grandmother took me into her house while I found somewhere to live, and my father helped me with part of the rent when I found a place and household items, as my salary would not be enough. Antonella and my grandma helped me out with food shopping and washing my clothes in their place, as mine didn't have a washing machine—not in the apartment or in the building. I felt so grateful for their support. I didn't expect anything from them and for them to give me a hand was not only kind and generous but helped me stand up in a moment when I had been knocked down.

Soon after I started living alone, my boyfriend ended our relationship. I was very much in love, so in addition to losing my mom, losing my boyfriend of two years was very hard on me. I lost twenty pounds in one month and immersed myself in my new job as a way to cope with my broken heart. Becoming the nerd was my only way to cope years ago. Then I became a workaholic for the rest of my working life.

It was a difficult time in my life, but one that I dedicated myself to overcoming. I learned a lot coming out of this experience and used it to become a strong, independent, self-sustaining woman. My family (both my father's and mother's side) had a wealthy life in Colombia and we were brought up with a lot of luxuries: belonging to private clubs; living in a big house, with maids, nannies, and a chauffeur; attending private schools and colleges; and enjoying sports and vacations abroad. That life ended suddenly as my mom kicked me out and I was still in the process of rebuilding my relationship with my father.

I had only started my internship in marketing at Frito-Lay, which barely covered my expenses. The apartment I rented was in a poorer area in the city, beside many prostitutes. It was safe enough and close enough to my office and friends, but it was clearly not in the same kind of neighborhood I was used to hanging around. I would not have enough money to go to the cinema and sometimes not even enough for groceries.

For that first year, I paid my bills using my credit cards and piling those credit-card bills one on top of the other. Ah! One thing I did buy was my first-ever cat. I was feeling so lonely, abandoned by the people who once used to love me, that I bought a gorgeous white Persian cat. I had it for three months and then it died! I cried my eyes out. It was so hard to lose him as he was my companion. He was born with a defective heart, so the pet store gave me another one as a replacement. So my second cat, which was identical to the first one, again lasted only three months! This time, I think it had a Superman complex and it thought it could fly. The apartment was on the thirteenth floor. When I arrived home, Tito was nowhere to be found. I had left a window open that was very high. I never thought she could reach it—two dead cats in seven months. I cried so much that I couldn't imagine getting another one. If something were to happen to it again, I couldn't deal with the sadness of it anymore. I now had even more reason to dig myself into work.

The experience of not having enough money even for groceries made me a hardworking woman. I also learned how to manage my finances in a smart, calculated way. Save, save and save. When I didn't have enough to save ten dollars a month, I tried to save five dollars. I am an independent woman, and my plan was to be so for the rest of my life. Knowing how difficult it is to live life by the penny or by credit card, I learned that I didn't want to ever have to feel that way again. I was so desperate and stressed every time I received a bill.

Not only did I learn this valuable lesson but I also learned that money does not give you happiness. Once I became strong again, I started living as happily without a penny as I had been before. With or without money, happiness is the same! It's the same feeling and the same amount, if you could quantify happiness.

After I finished my internship at Frito-Lay, they hired me immediately as a full-time employee. It was the best work experience ever. I loved the brands (Lay's, Doritos, Cheetos, etc.), the company, the friends I made there, the fun I had, and the valuable marketing lessons I learned. I started out as an assistant brand manager and was promoted as junior brand manager. I was extremely passionate, worked extremely long hours because I wanted to, and worked the weekends as it had become a pleasure. I traveled at first around Colombia to more than ten cities I had never been to, as my family normally vacationed outside of Colombia. I didn't do much international travel, with the exception of Venezuela, for work.

With the promotion, I was able to pay my expenses, but I earned just enough to do so. The office was one block from my dad's and Antonella's house, which became a great advantage because I could go home for lunch with them and also helped build my relationship with them further.

Marketing was my passion. I wanted to continue this path for the rest of my working career. I had a passion for multinational brands and the international aspect of them, which is aligned with my past. The biggest careers in marketing are always within the massive consumer goods sector and this was the arena I wanted to play in. I also wanted to be able to change industries, as I thought I would make my CV stronger by learning about different industries, strategies, and speeds within the industries. For people who don't work in marketing, there is much more to it than meets the eye. It is a highly strategic, analytical, and goal-oriented area of the company. I needed to be great in people-management skills as well as be financially oriented, as I would be responsible for the success of the brands, the brand equity, the profit and loss of the brands, return on investment, market-share value and sales in the market.

Building strong brands takes years and needs strong investments behind them, therefore working for them makes you part of their legacy.

Almost three years into this job, I was offered a job at Nokia (then the number-one mobile-phone company in the world—now it sounds like ancient history). The position paid more, enough that I would be able to save money, and also included a lot of international travel. Being twenty-six years old, single, and wanting to explore the world, it was a great opportunity.

And travel I did! I didn't spend more than one week in Colombia per month. During the year I worked with Nokia, I traveled several times to the United States, Venezuela, Jamaica, China, Brazil, Germany, Argentina and many more countries. The first seven months were great, but after so much travel, I became a bit of a loner. As I was never home, people assumed I wasn't there. They call in the beginning, but once they get repeated responses that I couldn't go out or see them because I was in another country, they stopped calling. The few times I was home, I saw family and then had to go away again. The lifestyle definitely made it difficult to have a relationship. Regardless, I enjoyed discovering new countries and being independent. I was a strong, young, happy working woman. It was a dream come true, and I wanted to continue dedicating my life to work and the happiness it gave me.

My life plan had always included getting an MBA, mostly because I wanted to continue to build a strong career for myself.

I had two specific criteria for choosing where to study:

1. I wanted it to be on the global top ten MBA list.
2. I wanted to be in a fun city to live in.

I opened the *Financial Times* 2007 top ten MBAs in the world and the MBA from IE Business School (Instituto de Empresas) was ranked eighth worldwide and second in Europe. It was in Madrid, Spain, a great, fun city. This was it. I applied to only this one MBA program, got accepted, quit Nokia, and was on my way to Madrid. It became the best year of my life. The name is not as famous as

Harvard or Wharton, but that's because they only have masters programs. They don't have undergraduate programs (at least, they didn't when I studied there), so the name is well known, but only among people who have completed MBAs.

The first seven months of the MBA program were long nights of studying, early alarms for finishing reading cases, and the Madrid nightlife! I made great lifelong friends during this year. The last months were a bit less stressful, and I had a bit more time to enjoy the city, friends, travel, and party. I sailed in two MBA sailing regattas as the captain of an eight-person boat in Portofino, Italy. Being surrounded by students from all across the world, with amazing years of work experience and different career backgrounds was the most amazing experience of my life. Most of the IE alumni describe that year as their best year in their lives.

I graduated from the MBA program in 2008. It wasn't easy to go back to a "normal life," where I was no longer surrounded by hundreds of friends from across the world. When I graduated, many students wanted to stay in Madrid, but the 2008 economic crisis hit. People couldn't find jobs in Spain, with its national unemployment rate of more than 25%, to they had to go back to their home countries. I was one of the only international students who found a job in Spain, so after my MBA, I stayed in Madrid.

I was actually blessed with three different job offers after my MBA: L'Oréal Spain, Johnson & Johnson (based out of Puerto Rico), and Alpina in Colombia. I chose L'Oréal, not only because it's a strong multinational with amazing brands but also because it would be the first time I would work in marketing in a developed country, which would enhance my learning for my career. For example, differences like getting daily Nielsen reports rather than monthly reports already made marketing significantly more mathematical and numbers based than when I had to create strategies with less-numerical information. In addition, Spain was the second-biggest market for the company, after France.

I worked in Garnier, part of the massive consumer-goods division with brands such as Garnier, L'Oréal Paris, and Maybelline, the most important division of L'Oréal. The other four divisions were luxury (with brands such as Lancôme, Giorgio Armani, Biotherm, Kiehl's, Yves Saint Laurent, Ralph Lauren, etc.), pharmacy (La Roche-Posay, Vichy, etc.), professional (Kérastase, Redken, Matrix, etc.), and the Body Shop.

My time there brought me great learnings, but even though I was a bit of a workaholic, L'Oréal took this to another level. I worked, on average, until at least nine pm, and three times a week until at least eleven pm. The company also had a strict French hierarchical culture and structure that didn't allow anyone's opinions. I had many friends who had worked for the company and advised me that the working atmosphere was terrible, but I ignored them, thinking, *It can't be that bad.* It was worse than I could possibly imagine! I hated it from day one. My work colleagues were nice, but the culture was terrible. You had no decision power and even the smallest decisions, like a sticker design, would need two layers of approval. A very strong micromanagement style. I decided to stay one year to learn, but not a day more. When I finally quit, it was one of my happiest days! I walked around with the biggest smile on my face, celebrating that I was leaving.

Johnson & Johnson called me again for the role they had offered me a year before. They still hadn't filled that position and really wanted me to take it. It was a regional role for Central America and the Caribbean Islands, based out of San Juan, Puerto Rico. It was a big change in a very different industry, but for a great company, with an important salary increase, and, best of all, living on a beach in the Caribbean while still advancing my career. Perfect!

I could not believe my view would be perfect blue ocean.

Sandals, flip-flops, sand and sunscreen. I loved it! It was a calm life compared to the big-city life I had always lived, which brought a lot of peace. I loved my boss and work colleagues and enjoyed the job. I went inline skating at night on the ocean front and bought my dream car, an Audi TT (which I called MosquiTTo). It had been my dream car for many years and I was so excited on the day I bought it that I arrived, like an idiot, two hours before the dealer opened just to look at it through the window. Driving was a passion of mine and now I had a superfast car. I bought a radar detector so I could speed and avoid the fines.

I didn't have time for relationships. They were not my priority. So the last official boyfriend I had was back in college.

Remember my mother was from Puerto Rico? My working there was completely independent of that fact, but, coincidently, when I started living in Puerto Rico, my mom remarried a Puerto Rican named Paco, and was spending time on the island. She introduced me to my Puerto Rican family, whom I had never met, and we also started spending a little more time together. We were both open to trying to make our relationship better. It was difficult and painful, but I was open to at least giving it a try.

Paco was a key person who opened that space and sharing moments with them made it easier than if it had been only her. He is such a kind, genuine, good person. My mom always finds the best men out there. I have to admit that.

Since I started speaking with my mom again, our relationship started to get significantly better. It's not like it was before "that sad night," and I'm not sure it will ever be, but I have 100 percent forgiven her. I'm looking forward to having something close to what I had with her before. I have to give her credit that she has tried nonstop to rebuild the relationship with me and has been kind, generous, and loving with me. The most important aspect is to allow the relationship to rebuild itself, and it will flow again naturally.

While living in Puerto Rico, I was approached by Diageo for a regional role: Central America and Caribbean luxury-brands marketing manager. Now that was a sexy role! Diageo, a British company, is the biggest spirits multinational in the world. You probably haven't heard the name, but for sure you have heard of its brands (Johnnie Walker, Smirnoff, Baileys, Captain Morgan, Tanqueray, Guinness, Captain Morgan, etc.). I would be in charge of the luxury portfolio, which included Johnnie Walker Blue Label, Johnnie Walker Platinum Label, and Johnnie Walker Gold Reserve, Ketel One, CÎROC, Tanqueray No. Ten, Tequila Don Julio and Zacapa Rum, among others.

The role involved heavy traveling, but I loved it because after a long week's work, I traveled back home, and home was like going on a vacation—a Caribbean island! Managing the luxury brands, I also traveled and visited luxury hotels and restaurants across the region. How could I possibly complain? I planned events on private yachts, in art museums and in polo clubs. I worked long hours and many weekends, but I loved it more than any job in my life. Work gave me 100% happiness. No need for anything else. I worked long hours because I was so passionate and loved it so much. I just wanted to. I didn't have to.

I often traveled to the United States, Europe, and South America for global meetings and/or events. Again, like at Nokia, I wasn't spending more than a week per month at home. I met Enrique and Sergio, my best friends in Puerto Rico. They were everything a girl needs! They were a gay couple, married for more than ten years. Enrique was a marketer like me and Sergio was a psychologist. How could I possibly need anyone else? Beach, friends, and work I loved. Great times. I was lucky in life, happy, and not expecting that I could be even happier soon!

I had been working with the man of my dreams for about a year, even though I didn't yet know it would be him. One year into my job at Diageo, two international people were relocated from the English office to the Puerto Rican office: a Brit (Simon) and a Greek (Tasos). Simon arrived from England with his French girlfriend and the four of us quickly became friends as we were all expats.

Simon and his girlfriend had been together for many years before arriving on the island, but it didn't quite work out well, as she went back to Europe two months after arriving in Puerto Rico. The remaining three of us continued hanging out together, both at work and outside of work. I was actually Simon's dotted-line manager.

It was not love at first site at all with Simon. I fell in love long after meeting him. In the beginning, I wasn't clear about the company policy about our relationship, so we quietly dated for a bit in silence. I also wanted to see if the relationship was worth making public or not. I won't write down the exact dates, as I know Tasos will be reading it to see if I wrote the true version here. To make Tasos even more curious, I won't, as he has never known the real version and is still dying to know. He has created so many scenarios in his head, so I'm going to allow him to continue inventing different answers to the same question. The only truth I will write is that we officially shared the relationship when we knew it was a serious one. The gossip will remain gossip.

Simon is the most romantic, generous, and kind man I had ever been with. He proposed to me in Virgin Gorda, with a bottle of champagne, a Cartier diamond ring, kneeling on the white sand of a perfect beach. I was so nervous and had never thought of what to answer if he ever proposed that the first thing that came to mind was, "Do I say thank you?"

I mean, he was giving me a ring, no? A gift? Ha-ha. Of course, I also said yes, but that was the first answer that came up,

"Do I say thank you?"

That night he took me to a surprise private dinner on the beach. The following day he rented a boat with a captain, and we sailed all day long. I can't stop smiling while I write this down. If only I could stop time, rewind the same day, and live it all over again and again. I would do that day and the day of our wedding, one year after he proposed. It was the happiest day of my life.

I couldn't imagine how happy I could be on my wedding day. The combination of marrying the man of my dreams, plus having all our friends and family together in the same place at the same time, made me happy like I had never imagined. We were married in Bogota, in the Country Club of Bogota (one of the ones my family belongs to). We had three bands thorough the wedding, a French one, a Latin one, and a DJ with an amazing singer for rock, so people from all cultures could enjoy the night. The wedding started at six in the evening and ended at five in the morning. Simon sang a song for me that he had composed and melted all women at the wedding. So romantic! We slept in Bogota for one night so we could relax before our exciting honeymoon and then off we were for the best month ever. We mixed a perfect combination with summer, beach, city, snow, and skiing! We started by staying one night in the W Hotel in South Beach, Miami, followed by Paris for one week to enjoy the city, opera, ballet, and romantic restaurants.

Then we took a train to Switzerland for a week of skiing in Zermatt, a pedestrian-only town in the mountains, with its iconic renowned Matterhorn peak (the one featured on Toblerone chocolate). We rented a Swiss chalet, a renovated old sheep barn in the oldest street of the town, remodeled with all the luxuries including a sauna, just for the two of us. We ate a lot of Swiss fondue and tons of Swiss chocolate, drank champagne every day on the terrace, and skied nonstop. We had perfect weather and the perfect mixture of snow and sun. All the pounds I lost for the wedding came back on quickly on this honeymoon. It was simply amazing!

We then took the train again, this time to the airport to fly to the Maldives! After perfect snow, we deserved some perfect beach. We stayed a full week in a water bungalow in a five-star resort on one of the picture-perfect islands. We had a private pool in the middle of the ocean in the bungalow for ourselves in the honeymoon suite. We woke up every morning to look at the fish through the glass below our feet in the bedroom and shower, had a quick dip in the flat, transparent-blue ocean, taking our private ladder down to the sea, and then headed off for breakfast.

When we couldn't take any more sun, we headed back to Paris to spend our first Christmas together as a married couple and bought our first Christmas tree. It was a drunken Christmas tree. No matter how hard we tried, it kept bending to one side. It looked like it had drunk more champagne than the liters we had drunk since the wedding day.

The last stop was New York City, to celebrate New Year's Eve and Simon's birthday.

It was the perfect honeymoon. We then returned to Miami. Yes, Miami and not Puerto Rico. Simon had received an offer within Diageo based out of Miami, and before starting our honeymoon we shipped all our stuff there from Puerto Rico. So when we came back, we were ready to start our life in Miami.

Within the first two months, we found the house we loved and bought our first home. It was less than a five-minute walk to Diageo, and since we both worked there, it was ideal. We had many issues with the house and had to invest in a lot of expensive projects like a new roof, but we loved it. We bought new furniture that fit perfectly in it. We dedicated months to decorating, repairing and filling our new home with love.

Tasos had also relocated to Miami at the same time, so "the Greek" continued to be close to us.

The Diageo CEO, who had been leading the company for thirteen years, left and was replaced. With a change in CEO came a big change in the company, leading with the biggest reorganization in years. With this, many positions were eliminated, especially from the areas of marketing and finance, and were replaced with sales positions. My and my teams' roles were eliminated. Many employees started looking for positions outside of Diageo as soon as they heard a reorganization was coming. I had a great offer on the table as marketing manager for the United States at Millicom, was a great career move. By coincidence, it was in the same building and, therefore, still a short walk from our new home.

Life was going great. At thirty-four, I was earning a six figure salary, living in our new home, in love, healthy, and enjoying life. I knew what it was to not have a penny; I knew what it was to not have enough for groceries; and, after ten years of working long hard hours, with dedication and passion, I was finally enjoying a successful career. I had one goal: to make it even better and even more successful. If I ever became a mom, my passion for my work meant I would want to continue as a working mom and work on building my career even further. I was a great wife with a great career, and, someday, I would be a great working mom. All the stars were aligned. I was also having a great relationship with every member of my family. It was a complete, fulfilled, and happy life. A perfect one! Nothing could possibly go wrong. Nothing could possibly change this happy path.

CHAPTER FIVE

REDISCOVERING LIFE

Home sweet home after my surgery. I was back to my world, my home, my bedroom, and my kitchen. Antonella had prepared a delicious lunch for me that day. I walked through the door to find my house full of flowers and gifts from my friends, work colleagues, and family. Flowers! I had never enjoyed flowers as much as I did that day. I was mesmerized by their beauty, their fresh, perfumed scent. They were a miracle of life. I know this might sound exaggerated, but I am being completely honest. I can't explain how much I was enjoying the flowers. I didn't understand the effect that the beauty in flowers caused in my brain.

I started a heavy routine of around eight different types of pills. Now that I no longer had the pleasure of the morphine to help with the pain, taking the drugs was the key making it bearable. There were so many pills that we laid them out in a dedicated space with instructions and times for each one so that Simon and Antonella could help me with them. Alone, it wouldn't have been possible—remember, I couldn't read or write. Having to take the pills by myself would have been impossible. It's amazing how useless we are without reading capabilities. I couldn't read a clock; I couldn't understand what taking a pill at three o'clock meant. The simplest things became impossible to do.

The pills were important for pain, avoiding infections, and most importantly, avoiding strokes. Strong steroids didn't let me sleep. Thinking that being sick means I would at least get to rest was far from the truth. The steroids had the side effect of insomnia. I fell asleep at eleven, and I would be awake from two until seven in the morning. I fell asleep again from seven to nine. Every single night. It was so boring with everyone asleep. All I could do was lie there, as I couldn't read or even watch TV, as the light was so bright I couldn't stand it and walking unaided at this point was not possible.

For the first time in my life, I was completely dependent on people. I was 100% dependent! I could not be alone in the house for the first month. I was so lucky that Simon got permission to work from home for the first month and a half to be able to help me out. Antonella and my dad helped me enormously as well, and my mom also came two weeks after my surgery to help me. I did not take this help for granted. Now that I am able to think and understand everything, I realize how lucky I was to have had this procedure near people who could help me 100%. I couldn't have done this by myself or living alone. I admire anyone who could do this alone. It is impossible!

For the first two months, I was unable to cook anything. I was so simpleminded, so dumb, I couldn't turn off the stove. I could have burned myself or started a fire. That is how scrambled my brain was! Using a knife would have been irresponsible as well, so I couldn't cut anything with a sharp knife.

Having lost my peripheral vision, getting around the house was difficult for the first couple of months. I stumbled on everything. I almost fell down the stairs and that was scary as my scar was still very fresh. So I decided not to use the stairs anymore.

I couldn't even take a shower myself for the first month. Antonella jumped into the shower with me in her bathing suit and washed my hair while I sat in a special plastic shower chair we bought before the surgery. I wasn't sure I would use it before the surgery, but, oh, what a smart decision it was to buy this chair in advance. We also had to dry my hair after the shower, as keeping it wet wasn't good for the scar, so Antonella, my mom, or Simon helped me. So much love!

I was rediscovering how to move, walk, and be around my own home. It was a fascinating period of rediscovering life. I rediscovered things, people, and feelings I would have never imagined I would rediscover.

Coloring was the only fun activity I could do, and how fun it was! How simple could my brain be that coloring like a two-year old was my favorite activity. Fun, fun, fun! I have never been artistic. I've always been business-driven and have never been curious about any form of art. It reflected the simplicity of the little child's brain that I had at that period of my recovery. I imagine it was shocking for my loved ones to see that the only activity I enjoyed was being with them or coloring. I was reliving life like a two-year-old.

I colored for days and hours, listening to classical music. I have always enjoyed classical music, but boy did I adore it at that time. It sounded like music from heaven. All other music sounded like horrible noises. I couldn't stand anything else. Fascinating how the brain relaxes with classical music, and how shocked it is with anything different.

For the first month, watching TV was so lame. Boring! First of all, I couldn't stand the light of the TV. But most importantly, I couldn't follow a program. I couldn't understand anything. Therefore, I didn't miss it. In modern society, TV plays such an important part of our daily routines for information and for pleasure. And here I was, with a lot of free time to enjoy TV and catch up on all those movies and series I hadn't had the time to watch when I was working, and I found them so boring I didn't watch any of it.

Rediscovering food was a life-changing experience. I have struggled with my weight my entire life, like many women do. I have been chubby for 70% of my life. As I am only five feet, I blamed it on my height, but we all know it was an excuse for not exercising enough and not eating properly to maintain a healthy weight. The other 30 percent of my life, I was slim. Having tasted being slim was the tipping point on my weight obsession. I was never satisfied with my weight. I've been on all the existing diets, paid the yearly membership to the gym to only go for one month, and blamed the weight gain on constipation and any other excuse I could find to make myself feel better.

Deep inside, I knew that they were all excuses and I lacked the will to manage the problem correctly or simply enjoy how I looked and accept myself. Since the brain surgery, something fascinating occurred to me, which linked to the simplicity of my brain! After the surgery, the only food that tasted good—and not only good, but great—were simple, natural foods. My brain was back to its basic instincts were vegetables, fruits, eggs, and organic meat (chicken, fish, pork, or beef) tasted amazing. Any processed food tasted horrible or like cardboard.

Most of what we eat these days has been filled with chemicals, mixes of ingredients, and new flavors that the basic palate does not recognize. All the new things we eat now are acquired tastes. For example, burgers, sauces, fried chips, French fries, pizza, and so on did not taste good at all. My body only wanted natural foods. It has now been nine months since I weighed forty-nine kilograms and have not gained a pound since. It's been effortless. No diet for the first time in my life! Unbelievable. This is how I truly understood the difference between healthy eating and not eating healthy. I have always known the theory, but for the first time in my life, my simple brain has chosen simple food, and I have kept it as my go-to food.

The only exception to this change was candy. The effect on the brain is probably the most eye-opening of all. It tasted delicious from the first moment but the effect amazed me. With a small chocolate or a couple of gummy bears (which I love), my energy levels went through the roof! I went on an ultimate high. It was funny: a thirty-four-year-old woman jumping up and down with some sugar. Well, keeping me happy was an easy task.

Rediscovering nature was a beautiful experience. We are so used to nature and its beauty that we take it for granted. It almost disappears from our eyes when we see it in our daily lives. I had the luxury of enjoying nature like little children do, but as an adult. We took short walks around the neighborhood and around the golf course at sunset, when I could stand the light, and I heard birds from a distance and stopped every step or two to admire them. I was so happy. Little birds everywhere. It was like I was seeing them for the first time in my life! I was mesmerized by the beauty and chirps of even ugly brown birds. It was fascinating how much I enjoyed any animal and any tree I passed. Those first walks took ages as I stopped at every natural spectacle.

My walks were short in the beginning as I got exhausted but little by little, we added a block to make them longer. I was always accompanied by someone, as crossing a street was dangerous at this stage.

While I was enjoying the beautiful sounds of nature, I also hated the strangest new ones in my head. The "crack-crack" was driving me crazy! My skull was falling into place again and healing, creating new bone in the area where they cut a lid. It constantly made a "crack-crack" noise. It would wake me up. Oh, what a freaky and annoying noise this was. In the beginning, it was impossible for my family to imagine until Simon finally heard it. It took some months for this noise to cease, so I had to learn to be patient and live with it.

I've had tinnitus since I was eighteen, which feels like a ringing in your ears after the noise of a nightclub. It drove me insane after the surgery. I couldn't sleep. It felt like I had been in a nightclub all day and every night. With my insomnia on top of that, it was really driving me crazy! It was so loud. But there was nothing we could do about it. These were some of the most annoying side effects of the surgery. Of course there was the pain, so I stuck to my painkillers as my only option.

Sensitivity to noises was difficult to manage. We all spoke at very low levels as I couldn't handle. I could only walk the streets when there were no noises around.

Being so simpleminded or, in other words, having a brain that was close to that of a small girl, brought new traits. One of the strongest was the complete loss of hypocrisy. They say children don't know how to lie and are therefore honest about what they say and feel. I was also completely incapable of lying and, most importantly, of being a hypocrite to people I didn't really care about. It was powerful to be so close to my true feelings about the people I cared about and the people who deep down in my heart, I don't. This realization made me honest and truly appreciative of the people I loved.

One month after the surgery, I started the long path to recovery with cognitive therapy. It was strange to go to a hospital for this. It was difficult as I couldn't drive, so my husband had to take me every time. He worked on his laptop in the car while I attended my one-hour a week therapy.

In the beginning, we focused on simple things, like drawing a clock and putting the times on it. It was so difficult! Putting four-fifteen, for example, took me ten minutes to figure out. Problem-solving was also difficult. For example, if I need to be at an appointment at 10:20 a.m. and need to leave forty minutes before to get there on time, when do I need to leave? It was impossible for me. I had to break it down into several steps.

Communication was difficult. As I couldn't read or write for the first two months after the surgery, I had to use new tools. WhatsApp voice messages came as a lifesaver for communication. Even though I told my friends and family that I couldn't read or write, they still sent me e-mails, WhatsApp messages, and so on, which I then had to get my husband to read for me.

I also took homework to do therapy at home. My therapist kindly gave me a copy of the therapy book she used so that I could advance at home if I wanted to. This became my new day-to-day. I did therapy at home all day long. Everything in the first months was therapy because everything was so difficult.

My memory was short term. If somebody read five words to me, I could only remember one or two. Every family member who visited me during the first months helped me to do therapy by reading some words to me and I tried to remember them.

Therapy would be my full-time job for the next several months. I remember how difficult everything was.

Two months in, my husband had to start working from the office again. This was around the time I started to be able to read and write better. I still flipped letters. So instead of writing a lowercase *b*, I wrote *d*. It was strange because in my head, I knew I wanted to write a word like *desk*, but my hand wrote *besk*. Even on the computer, I typed *b* instead of *d*.

Speaking was also difficult. I got stuck all the time. Words wouldn't come out of my mouth. It was difficult to find the words I needed to be able to speak. It was the lack of words and what I described as the cat-hairball effect. Like when a cat chokes on a hairball, even if I knew what I wanted to say, I choked, and the words just didn't come out. It was very frustrating. The only thing I could do was breathe, relax, be more patient, and try again.

Therapy in the United States was expensive. Even with the insurance, the copay for one hour's therapy was sixty dollars. So three months into therapy, my dad and Antonella invited me to Colombia and paid for one month of intensive therapy there. In a specialized recovery group for brain and physical therapy, I attended speech and cognitive therapy for three hours daily. It was tiring, but it was definitely important for my recovery.

The trip was difficult. My husband couldn't travel with me (although he did join me in Colombia a couple of weeks later), and so I had to travel alone. I couldn't even understand how to get to a gate. Being around so many people, my only desire was to be invisible. I felt so nervous, as if I had never flown in my life. Believe me, I've flown to all the continents for work and for pleasure, and I lived in different places. Traveling was *not* an issue for me. But this time, I felt like a six-year-old having to travel alone. I required assistance and a wheelchair, both in the departure airport and the arrival.

The person sitting beside me on the airplane was a kind man around my age. He was doing some complex mathematical equations in a notebook. I asked him about what he was doing and he explained that he was a mathematician who had graduated from

MIT and was traveling to Universidad de los Andes, which is the college I graduated from in Colombia, to give a lecture to students there. We were probably the smartest and dumbest people on the plane. Here I was sitting with an MIT genius, and I couldn't even add four plus five. At the end of our stay in Colombia, I got to go with Simon to our ultimate favorite place called Mesa de Yeguas, a private country club, set amongst the mountains, overlooking a lake and lush green trees, for some sun and rest. I was especially happy that Simon got to rest, because it had been three intense months of having to work, not resting, and having a disabled wife he had to do everything for.

When we came back to Florida, we had our follow-up appointment with Dr. Smith. This was probably the most shocking appointment of all. Every time we saw him, the expected recovery date was always pushed back. We started with a three-week recovery, and then six-weeks. After this visit with him, the new window was six months from the surgery. That was a shocker, as he said we didn't really even know about the six-month recovery time.

For the first time, I burst into tears. So far everything had been fun coloring and amazing morphine and enjoying being stupid, but only because I thought it was short term. As it was temporary, I would enjoy every single phase of my simple brain, but wait six months like this? What about my job? I had signed up for the possibility of the peripheral eyesight loss, but I hadn't signed up for cognitive deficits.

Dr. Smith said that he expected the peripheral eyesight to come back by now, but, just in case, six months after surgery we would do an MRI with DTI to check if the nerves were intact.

I went back home with Simon. We were sad and shocked. After crying for a day or two, I pulled myself together, and there I went again. Intensive therapy time. Time to get better. There was one thing I knew for sure. I would do everything I could to avoid permanent cognitive deficits. So I continued daily therapies, and I called a psychologist to vent because this news was not expected. And I started what would be my routine for the next months:

- 2:00–5:00 a.m.: Insomnia (grr…but there was nothing to do about it)
- 5:00–8:30 a.m.: Recover from insomnia
- 8:30–9:00 a.m.: Eat fruit for breakfast
- 10:00–11:00 a.m.: Go to gym with a trainer. Why the gym? Even though it wasn't really a therapy I needed, I was willing to do everything I could. You know the saying: healthy body, healthy mind. So yes, gym it was for me.
- 11:00 a.m.–12:30 p.m.: Shower after gym and a healthy lunch
- 12:30–6:00 p.m.: Nonstop therapy.

Human resources and my boss were also expecting an update on my recovery process after my trip to Colombia and the visit I had with Dr. Smith. They asked me to come in with Simon, so we went together. It was easy anyway, as Simon's office was in the same building as mine. So we went directly to the HR floor, which was one floor higher than the floor with all my colleagues (which I preferred, as I was not psychologically ready to see them).

We arrived in a meeting room with one HR person and Adam. I don't remember the details of the meeting because early into it, I received the news that they had to let me go. I was so shocked that the meeting became a blur. Simon was there, so he could retain the information, because I left that meeting with one only memory: *Shit! I just got fired because of a brain tumor.* It was a double punch in one week. Now I really needed that psychologist.

I went home and cried a lot. Simon, like always, was an angel and a great support to me. In the United States, it's legal to let an employee go after three months of sick leave and it had been four months at that point. So they could legally let me go. And honestly, I have no bad feelings at all. On the contrary, they were kind from day one, and I am grateful to them and especially Adam. Millicom were generous with their patience and their compensation while I was sick. Many companies wouldn't have helped out at all and Millicom were great.

In the meeting, I couldn't stop my tears. While I did have tears, they were of sadness because I didn't understand how all this happened, from a short "three weeks off" to losing my job because I was still unable to work. I was just so sad and confused about my situation, but I remember that I couldn't stop thanking them for their kindness and support through the process. So I had mixed feelings, both genuine. Thank you, Millicom, and thank you, Adam and Teddy, for the support you gave me. I will be eternally grateful for it!

After this meeting, I was worried about my doctors and health insurance. I lost my health insurance and had to change to Simon's and make sure the doctors and therapists I was seeing were still covered. The copays were different, but at least I could continue seeing the same people.

A new worry started kicking in with the loss of my job— money and our mortgage. I had two months left of the short-term disability, which covered 60 percent of my salary. Knowing that my condition could last more than six months, I had to apply for long-term disability with the insurance and Social Security long-term disability. It took many weeks with Simon's help to gather all the papers we needed to send with the application. It took six months to get an answer.

We stopped receiving the disability checks six months after the surgery, and our economic situation changed completely. We had to start making important financial decisions. Unfortunately for us, we lost the higher salary. With only Simon's salary, we were unable to cover the fixed costs of the house and medical bills. We had to review our finances, made significant changes to our lifestyle, and also received help from my family so we wouldn't lose our house. But these changes would only help the problem for the short term.

If I couldn't work in the near future, we would have to make bigger decisions and sell the house and move into a significantly cheaper location. Again, why did all this happen to me? To us? Because this was also happening to Simon. At this point, we decided to wait three to four more months and see how the recovery was going before making the final decision to sell our house.

The next two months were based on the routine I shared earlier and I received visits from my sisters. I also started seeing some friends from Diageo and Millicom and went out for lunch with them to places that were within walking distance, which gave my days some variety and also forced me to go out a little and feel less nervous. First, crossing the street was a big deal, so I tried to cross two the next time, and so on until I could walk the Miracle Mile by myself (still feeling nervous but at least doing it). And yes, I was still crying from time to time about how confusing this situation was.

Encounters were better with fewer people. Simon once took me to a BBQ with some Diageo friends of his, whom I knew from my previous job, but being with more than fifteen people was a psychological shock for me. It was too difficult to manage. It broke me. We had to leave early as I really couldn't manage it. Even now, I still feel the emotional pain I went through because I wasn't ready to see people (no one's fault, as I had accepted to go, I just didn't realize that I wasn't ready).

I couldn't drive yet, but I did start to ride a bicycle with a helmet on to the gym. Driving, obviously, was out of question.

I started watching TV again with a low volume. I only watched animal documentaries—I was mesmerized by them. I still couldn't follow a movie or series, but, little by little, I was finally able to do what all working people do when they're sick: catch up on all the series that they hadn't have the time to watch. So yep…I watched them all! Not that I was super smart yet, but at least I could understand basic TV programs.

In May, I finally got back on social media, at first just with some pictures and Simon helping me write. It's interesting how we spend hours of our lives looking at Facebook and all sorts of social media and news, and as soon as I couldn't read or write, I completely lost interest. So I didn't check any of it for a long time. In addition, I didn't really want to share much of my personal life. When I did start sharing, it was only some pictures—nothing that would give a clue about what had happened to me or what I was going through.

I was lucky that the supermarket was one block away. I went back to food shopping. Simon did this for months after the surgery. I only got what I could carry, but at least I was helping out with the home necessities. I also started washing some clothes at home, but I was careful of the two steps that I had already almost fallen from many times. Falling down two steps! It's like drowning in a puddle. But yes, that was my adventure: trying not to fall down a two-step entrance to my garage.

Four or five months after the surgery, I could read and understand a bit more, so I went into an obsessive research phase to try to understand what had happened to me. I went into the surgery absolutely ignorant about what I had, other than what the doctor had told me. Now, seeing so many side effects that were never mentioned to me, I wanted to understand every single detail: what specific tumor I had, therapies I could do, and so on. I learned all the details about the intraventricular meningioma and the peripheral eyesight loss I had suffered from.

These are brain tumor statistics from the American Brain Tumor Association:

- Nearly 78,000 new cases of primary brain tumors are expected to be diagnosed this year. This figure includes nearly 25,000 primary malignant and 53,000 nonmalignant brain tumors.
- It is estimated that more than 4,600 individuals between the ages of 0–19 will be diagnosed with a primary brain tumor this year.
- There are nearly 700,000 people in the United States living with a primary brain and central nervous system tumor.
- This year, nearly 17,000 people will lose their battle with a primary malignant and central nervous system brain tumor.
- Survival after diagnosis with a primary brain tumor varies significantly by age, medical history, molecular markers, and tumor behavior.
- The median age at diagnosis for all primary brain tumors is 59 years.
- Meningiomas represent 36.4% of all primary brain tumors, making them the most common primary brain tumor. There will be an estimated 24,880 new cases in 2016.[4]

It goes on to describe meningioma as follows:

> Meningiomas usually grow inward, causing pressure on the brain or spinal cord. They also can grow outward toward the skull, causing it to thicken. Most meningiomas are noncancerous, slow-growing tumors. Some contain sacs of fluid (cysts), mineral deposits (calcifications), or tightly packed bunches of blood vessels.

[4]American Brain Tumor Association. (2016). Retrieved from http://www.abta.org/about-us/news/brain-tumor-statistics/.

Symptoms: Meningiomas usually grow slowly, and may reach a large size before interfering with the normal functions of the brain. The resulting symptoms depend on the location of the tumor within the brain. Headache and weakness in an arm or leg are the most common symptoms. However, seizures, personality changes, and/or visual problems may also occur.

Incidence: Meningiomas account for about 36.1% of all primary brain tumors, which are tumors that form in the brain or its coverings. They are most likely to be found in adults older than 60; the incidence appears to increase with age. Rarely are meningiomas found in children. They occur about twice as often in women as in men.[5]

There are many types of meningiomas with very different symptoms and probabilities of occurrence. Below are the different types and the percentage corresponding to each type.

---

[5] American Brain Tumor Association. (2016). Retrieved from http://www.abta.org/brain-tumor-information/types-of-tumors/meningioma.html?referrer=https://www.google.com/.

- Falx and parasagittal - 25%
- Convexity - 20%
- Sphenoid wing (also called sphenoid ridge) - 20%
- Olfactory groove - 10%
- Suprasellar - 10%
- Posterior fossa - 10%
- Intraventricular - 2%
- Intraorbital - <2%
- Spinal - <2%

[6]

I had one of the rarest, called intraventricular meningioma, which account for only 2 percent of all the meningiomas. I almost won the lottery except, instead of money, I got a brain tumor. I was younger than average to get them.

What was fascinating to me, was that I didn't realize I was having side effects. Headaches. I had daily headaches that were so bad I would carry Tylenol with me religiously. I just put this down to, too much computer time, work stress or not enough water. Very common to my brain tumor, and something I failed to notice.

---

[6] Brain Science Foundation. (2016). Retrieved from https://www.brainsciencefoundation.org/brain-tumor-resources/meningioma/locations/

CHAPTER SIX

FROM ABOVE AVERAGE TO BELOW AVERAGE

By August 2015, six months had passed since the surgery. I felt I had made many improvements since the first day out of surgery, but many were still to be made. I was clearly not even close to feeling normal. When would I feel normal again? One more month? Two? Six? In my mind, I would be normal again after a year, so I had six more months of this and that was it, back to normality. Or so I thought.

Unemployed and not knowing when I would be able to work again, I was starting to worry more about my future, although not too much as I was still looking forward to good news from Dr. Smith and my six-month MRI with DTI. I had also booked a visit with a neuro-ophthalmologist at Bascom Eye Institute at the University of Miami, who was ranked number one in the country. A month previously, I had a first appointment with a neuropsychologist, a specialty I didn't know existed. According to healthline.com website, "A neuropsychologist is a physiologist who specializes in understanding the relationship between the physical brain and behavior. The brain is extremely complex, and disorders within the brain or nervous system can alter behavior and cognitive function."[7]

I had been recommended to see a Neuropsychologist for my cognitive deficits. When I saw him for the first time, he gave me a long cognitive and IQ test that took more than six hours. The place looked like a normal doctor's office. The test was done both on paper and computer. The computer was very old. It reminded me of the ones we used to use at school, complete with a 5.35 floppy disc. It would take one month to get the results, so I was looking forward to them. It would be a big month. From this, I was hoping to get a lot of good news!

Going into the MRI machine felt like "home"—not in a good way, but in a such-a-familiar-feeling way. Simon took me to the appointment, and, this time, the MRI took longer as I had the DTI exam, which was interesting. It consisted of me having to open my eyes during the MRI so I could see a little screen inside the machine that passed many images at different speeds.

That same week, I got the results from my two doctors' appointments.

The "Monopoly man" (I'm not kidding—the doctor was an identical replica of Rich Uncle Pennybags) was a very nice doctor.

---

[7] Health Line. (2015). Retrieved from
http://www.healthline.com/health/neuropsychologist.

He also taught medical students, so they all looked at my case as it was interesting for them. He looked like a great teacher, too.

He made me do many exams that day. My eyesight was twenty/twenty. I also had peripheral eye exams there to compare with the ones I had done three months ago in Colombia to see if there were improvements. The exam consisted of me putting my head into a white machine and looking straight ahead, without moving my eyes. A little light turned on from time to time 180 degrees around me. When I saw the light, I clicked. After a long day of exams, from eight in the morning to four in the afternoon, and seeing the doctor, I had the results.

Since the exams in Colombia, there had been no change. It was still the same. Unfortunately, there is no medical treatment for this diagnosis as it is not the eyes but the brain that doesn't recognize that it can see. But I still wanted to check with Dr. Smith the day after, so my hopes were still up.

The one piece of good news after this visit was that I met the legal criteria for driving! I knew, though, that I couldn't see on the right side of both eyes, but I can drive on smaller streets during the day. So I started driving short distances with my husband, like to the supermarket, always taking small roads, never the highways. Miami is a tough place to drive for long distances, as many include big highways and required crossing many lanes to exit, so I was limited to where I could go and especially the time it would take me, but, for the moment, there was no stress as my hopes were still up.

Finally, it was time for the visit with Dr. Smith. It was nice to see him again. I don't know why, but every time I see him, I get a peaceful feeling. He is truly a great doctor and a gentle person who treats me well emotionally, as he seems to understand what his patients are going through.

He started his routine check and I could add and subtract, but multiplication was difficult (division was impossible). I could write, but slowly, and I read even more slowly as per my visual deficit. We looked at the MRI results, and the good news was that the tumor had been removed completely (which minimizes the possibility of it coming back). He showed me the scan. Instead of a tumor, I now had a big hole that looked like an upside-down cat. I asked him if the hole would close up with time, but he said it wouldn't, as the tumor was too big. Now I have a safety-deposit box in my brain! He also saw that the visual nerves were not affected after the surgery. Unfortunately, by now, six months after surgery and no visual nerves affected, he did not expect the peripheral vision to come back at all at this point.

After he examined me, he said that my recovery could take one year to eighteen months and there was a possibility that I would never be the same as before. Wait...*what*? Maybe never be the same again? What the hell! This was so shocking to me and Simon.

I had signed up for a 2% chance of losing my peripheral sight. From that to having strong cognitive deficits, maybe for life? To begin with, what were the chances of hitting that 2%? None! I also had Gerstmann syndrome that would affect me for life. Why was I not aware of this? Why was I not told about this possibility? I didn't want this possibility.

I wouldn't have signed up for the surgery if I had known that my cognitive brain—meaning my intelligence, everything that defines me, was at risk. I am not a hotshot; I am not a supermodel. The only things that defined me are my brain and my passion for work. I might never work again in the managerial marketing jobs like I had done before. *What? No! Fuck no.*

This time I did burst in tears in his office and so did Simon. We were not expecting this at all. Not even close. The possibility of this being permanent was never even a possibility in my mind. From not being a possibility to being a potential reality was heart-breaking. Dr. Smith was very kind and patient and waited for us to ask anything we wanted to and gave us some time to breathe.

We went home and I felt complete sadness for a week, but even so, I still had hope for the appointment with the neuropsychologist.

I was really looking forward to when the neuropsychologist's results were in. Unfortunately, Simon couldn't come with me that day. I knew the results were important and would give me a good picture of not only the reality but the before and after effects of the surgery. This is because eight months prior to my surgery, I participated in a job-interview process at SAAB Miller for the position of Latin American marketing regional manager. In the final phase of the process, they flew me to Chicago for a complete day of testing using a highly sophisticated IQ test, the Wechsler Adult Intelligence Scale—Fourth Edition (WAIS-IV).

According to Wikipedia, "The Wechsler Adult Intelligence Scale (WAIS) is an IQ test designed to measure intelligence and cognitive ability in adults and older adolescents. The original WAIS (Form I) was published in February 1955 by David Wechsler, as a revision of the Wechsler-Bellevue Intelligence Scale, released in 1939. It is currently in its fourth edition (WAIS-IV) released in 2008 by Pearson, and is the most widely used IQ test, in the world."[8]

The test was administered by an external company. I didn't get the results after the testing, as they were exclusively for SAAB Miller and the interview process, but after my surgery, I remembered I had the e-mail address and name of the outside

---

[8] Wikipedia contributors. " Wechsler Adult Intelligence Scale ". Wikipedia, The Free Encyclopedia. (2015). Retrieved from https://en.wikipedia.org/wiki/Wechsler_Adult_Intelligence_Scale.

company that gave the test to me. I wrote to them and explained what had happened and asked them if, as an exception, they could share my results with me so that I could compare what my IQ was before the surgery with the new results. They made the exception for me and sent them over. They even called me to go over the results.

"Nathalie Jacob, your full range IQ is 114, *high* average range."

I had completed the test in English, and, as it not my first language, the results would have been lower than if the test had been in Spanish, but the examination with the neuropsychologist was in English too, so the two tests would be comparable. The WAIS-IV IQ test was based on my age group and education level. According to Wikipedia, "Two broad scores, which can be used to summarize general intellectual abilities, can also be derived Full Scale IQ (FSIQ), and the General Ability Index (GAI),"[9] and my results in both were *above* average. My FSIQ was 114 (high average range), and my GAI 118 (high average range).

The neuropsychologist sat down with me for more than an hour and went over every single result of the test.

My IQ was 87, *below* average range. In his report, he wrote, "There is no question that the condition of this patient reflects a wide variety of impairments of higher cerebral functions estimated to be the sequela to the presence of a left hemisphere intraventricular meningioma occipital parietal meningioma."[10] Ouch! That hurt so very much. Below average!

---

[9] Wikipedia contributors. " Wechsler Adult Intelligence Scale ". Wikipedia, The Free Encyclopedia. (2015). Retrieved from https://en.wikipedia.org/wiki/Wechsler_Adult_Intelligence_Scale#Index_scores _and_scales.
[10] Neuropsychologist report, 2015, p. 10.

So that day I was in a dark place, that place in the tunnel where the slim light at the end completely disappeared. Below average! So now my neurosurgeon told me I may never return to normal. If that meant I would be like that for the rest of my life, did it mean I was below average? Jobless, dumb and unable to maintain myself for the rest of my life? That I would not be able to work ever again? When did all this happen to me? I felt like my world was falling apart.

This was the darker side. I needed to take action and make sad, long-term decisions. If I would not be able to work again—and not just work again, but work in the salary ranges I was in prior to my surgery—then I needed to make important, life-changing decision. It was so sad to even think about making changes in my happy life and the impact this would also have on Simon's life. We were a happy, in-love couple. We were successful and enjoying the "peak moment" of our careers and the luxuries that come with that, and, in the blink of an eye, the life we had planned and were living had completely changed.

We had bought our house a year ago and had just finished putting in the new pool and blinds, doing all the little things we loved. We bought the house based on our finances at the time. With both our jobs, we could pay the mortgage, and, if one of us ended up out of work, we could maintain it for a year. We never intended to have only one salary to maintain it, especially not for life. Even worse, it was the bigger salary that had disappeared. This was our new reality and we would have to start taking action.

We would not be able to cover the fixed costs anymore, including the mortgage, unless we received some help from my family. This would be a short-term solution. I called my realtor Ileana (whom I love, as she has been a great realtor, friend, and support since we met her in Miami) to understand what costs would be involved in selling our house, what the potential price would be if we were to sell, and if we would recover all that we had invested. If we couldn't, what could we rent the house for in order to minimize the losses while we sold it?

Indeed, it was too soon to sell it without losing the investment we made, so I started to look for places to rent so we could move out of the house. I looked at personal things to potentially start selling. We also had to make the sad decision to sell *Valentina*, my Valentine's gift from Simon the year we arrived in Miami: a new blue Vespa. It was still almost new as I hadn't been able to use it since the surgery. This was probably the hardest decision as I had a lot of affection for it.

We had to do a new household-income analysis and cut down every expense.

I immediately started the cognitive therapies at the neuropsychologist's office, going twice a week as he recommended. He also stated that he thought that I could improve with this therapy. So the fight was far from over.

On the other hand, the fight for the peripheral vision was basically finished. I had to start accepting my forever deficits. Honestly, it didn't bother me that much—at least compared to the cognitive deficits. It was not the end of the world at all. I could learn to adapt. Yes, I would miss many things, like sailing in competition, driving normally, sitting at a dinner table and being able to see the person at my right, not bumping into things and people I couldn't see and reading at a normal speed. At least I could compensate in terms of books by listening to them instead of reading them. Driving is one of the biggest losses. It does have its advantages! If I do want to ignore someone I can do so easily; I just need to put the person on my right side.

I also started experiencing new side effects for the first time.

Either I didn't have them before, or I didn't notice them because I thought they were temporary, as it was too close to the surgery. The biggest one and the one that was going to be one of the strongest ones for life was *brain fatigue*.

The most annoying part of this one is that "normal" people don't really believe or understand me. They think I am exaggerating or faking it, being lazy, or finding excuses by saying I am tired. But it is a completely different feeling. It's not the "I'm tired after a day's work" feeling when you get home. It's not a "tired" feeling at all. It's like my brain goes back months in recovery. It completely shuts down and I can't even add basic numbers. My brain is working much harder than a normal brain and it needs to recharge its batteries.

Early in the recovery, it was difficult to differentiate brain fatigue due to recovery from brain fatigue as a long-term side effect. I started noticing it on specific occasions where my routine changed, and, therefore, I risked brain fatigue. For example, my parents went to Palm Beach for a couple of weeks' vacation with my youngest sister, Marie, and passed through Miami to visit us. Simon and I went to Palm Beach to spend some time with them there. As I was able to hold conversations better than when we saw each other in Colombia, we spoke more and did more. I couldn't manage my energy levels. My brain fatigue immediately kicked in. They wanted me to go to the beach with them and I simply couldn't manage it, so I stayed in the apartment.

I couldn't really stand the sun either. It was too much for my eyes as I was more sensitive to light as well. I was nervous with my scar on my head too. Even though the nurse had said it would be fine in the ocean, I didn't want to risk any pain or getting sand near it. All this brain fatigue also made me grumpy. It was uncomfortable to be like this. I knew I was grumpy, and I apologized for being so, but I couldn't stop it. I did not enjoy the weekend at all. This side effect lasted maybe a month or two. Strange…but lucky it wasn't permanent. It affected my happiness and the people around me.

My husband had generously bought tickets for the Juan Luis Guerra concert in Miami. He's a famous Latin American merengue singer from the Dominican Republic whom I love. Simon had bought the tickets before the surgery and had them as a surprise. That surprise ended up being a nightmare for me. We went to the concert and I couldn't stand the volume. I took earplugs, but even with them, it was horrible. Being surrounded by thousands of people made me anxious as well. I hated it! It was impossible to enjoy and I was really tired, we left half way through.

One of the pleasures of going to a concert is singing along with the songs. But if you put earplugs in, all you hear when you sing is your own voice vibrations. It wasn't fun at all. So not singing and not being able to enjoy the music and being surrounded by crowds was a complete disaster for my new brain. I honestly think that will be the last time I go to a concert. I feel bad saying this because Simon loves concerts, but I doubt I will be able to ever go with him again.

Music has become too difficult for me to bear. I can only listen to classical music now. I have always loved it, but I have loved other types too. In the car with Simon and in the house, I can only listen to classical music or nothing at all. I feel bad for him because he loves many types of music, but I can't stand it. It's so unfair to him. I try to make the effort, but I cannot stand it. My brain can't!

Loud restaurants, loud bars…don't even mention nightclubs. I can't stand the noise anymore. Why doesn't my brain process them? I don't know. I don't understand, but it's annoying to not be able to, not only for me, but for the people around me. I hope these new side effects will disappear soon, because if not, I am the oldest thirty-four-year-old person in the world. Poor Simon. He married a fun, smart girl, and he has ended up with a boring, dumb one.

In September, Simon and I went to the wedding of one of my best friends in Colombia. Those weeks in Colombia were nice. I got to see family and spent my thirty-fifth birthday with them and friends.

Being at the wedding was strange for me. I was so anxious. Even though it was people I had known for years, and two of my best friends were there, I still felt nervous and uncomfortable. They were probably the only ones who knew about my situation, so I felt isolated because I didn't want to tell anyone else. When people came and asked me how I was and what was I up to these days, my answer was just, "Good, thank you. Living in Miami." I didn't engage in conversations longer than a minute. I was so nervous. I was stuck to my husband like chewing gum—I didn't want to let go! I was so anxious! It was strange. I don't know if the people around me noticed or not. I never asked and never will.

Hitting thirty-five filled me with mixed feelings. My grandmother arranged a lovely dinner at her house and invited my family and some good friends over and prepared her famous secret-recipe rum cookies, which we love. She only bakes them for special occasions and has never shared the recipe with anyone. I was happy for the opportunity to be with loved ones, but, at the same time, I was hitting an important age, when I was supposed to be at the peak of my professional career. Instead, there I was, unable to divide numbers. So it was indeed a happy day, but I shed some tears with my husband at the end of it, because life had given me a thirty-fifth birthday present I was not expecting.

Traveling this time was more manageable. I was nervous, but at least I could read numbers, so I got to go to the gates by myself and managed. What progress! I'm not saying that I felt normal, but at least I didn't need a wheelchair. It was an accomplishment.

Back in Miami, I continued my routine and started to go inline skating, which I have always done and loved. Simon gave me new blades for my birthday, so I was happy using them for the first time. This time around, I used a helmet because I didn't want to risk falling on my not-fully recovered skull.

As if life hadn't changed enough, Simon was offered a new role within the same company, but based out of Norwalk, Connecticut. It was a great professional next step for him in his career, but Connecticut was going to be more expensive than Florida at a time when his was the only salary. Now, share plans are great in the long term, but people don't eat shares or sleep on them. They don't pay medical bills either, which were our mailbox's favorite meal.

It was a difficult decision to make, one that gave me a lot of anxiety, but we needed to make some changes in our life anyway due to my job loss.

Coincidently, Simon's new boss from the Netherlands was relocating to Miami with his family at the same time that we were making our decision, and he was looking to rent a place. We showed him our house, which was not even a block from Diageo, and he loved it. He wanted to rent it immediately as he had only two more weeks in his temporary accommodations. So we had to decide immediately if we would rent the house out, move, and take the new role.

It was a tough decision. We were so happy in Miami and in our house with our new pool. But it seemed like destiny had arranged all this for a reason. We couldn't afford our house anymore anyway, so renting it out meant it would maintain itself. We finally made the decision by choosing between a bikini or a winter coat. Rationally, Connecticut was the decision to make. Emotionally, it was not what we wanted, but it was what our rational selves told us to do. If my brain tumor had not happened, we would not have moved out of Miami, as losing my salary would not have made sense at all, but given that I had already lost that, moving was a possibility in order to progress Simon's career.

In only two weeks we were out of our house and staying in a hotel for the last week in Miami. There was almost no time to say good-bye. Nothing.

I would have to continue with my therapies and doctors in the northeast, which we thought would be easier than in Miami. So we thought at the time…

In October, we left Miami.

CHAPTER SEVEN

THE NEW/ REST OF MY LIFE

We arrived at the temporary accommodation that was offered as part of the moving package Simon received. He also got a two-week car rental while our car arrived from Miami in a truck. The apartment was OK. It was a small one-bedroom in Stamford. It wasn't very pretty, but it did the job. It definitely wasn't a place to feel at home or to want to stay longer than needed.

While Simon started work immediately, I looked for houses to rent within the budget Simon set. Having one car was a bit of a hassle because nothing was within walking distance, and, in order for me to be able to move during the day, I had to drop Simon off and pick him up at work, which didn't help with my fatigue. Getting the second car was a priority, but, for that, I needed an address to get a lease.

The rental market was varied in the area. Most rentals came up entering the summer, but we were entering winter, and there were not many options out there. We thought that as I wasn't working and would spend most of my time in the house, finding one the approximate size of the one in Miami would be practical. That way, I wouldn't feel like I was in jail, and we could also fit all our furniture coming up, like our two sofas (we had two living rooms).

We saw over twelve houses and liked only one or two, but they were a bit out of our budget. We ended up renting the cheapest one we found that had the characteristics we needed. We didn't love it, but it was OK. It was near Simon's work in the Diageo headquarters (a ten-minute car ride), which would be an added value. Since I would spend all day alone, a short commute for him was key.

The house layout was OK but wasn't really our style, as we like modern, open spaces, and this house was individually spaced areas with strange decorations and colors. We also found it strange that the landlords gave us the house with a lot of nail holes and nails in every room, and it was dirty. I had to clean the shower six times before using it even once. Disgusting! There was a very old washing machine that I didn't think to check before. The other appliances were old and wasted energy. There were no LED bulbs whatsoever, but changing all the bulbs in the house would be expensive, so we kept the lights dimmed most of the time.

The neighborhood was nice though, even though the house was in Norwalk, it was across the street from New Canaan, a town with gorgeous houses with an average cost of $2 to $4 million. When we went out for walks, we walked in New Canaan, even though we paid Norwalk prices.

The leaves were already starting to fall, and winter was coming. I felt happy for the first month up north. It was so pretty.

The trees were full of orange, red, and yellow leaves. The weather was nice, and seeing the beautiful houses was a great experience.

We moved into the house in November, and, as Simon was working, I did all the unpacking, which took forever on my own. It was an exhausting task, especially since we had a big house and many items. It took me two complete weeks of unpacking. I really wanted to finish installing myself before getting into therapy and my routine again. So I dedicated myself to house tasks: setting up accounts, changing addresses, getting the Internet and TV installed, cleaning the house, and washing everything that we had moved from Miami. They were never-ending, boring tasks. We hadn't found the gardeners yet, so we had to pick up all the leaves after they fell, and that took hours without the proper tools.

Moving is definitely not fun. The older you get, the more you hate it. I've moved so many times to different countries and apartments—on average, more than once every two years for the past ten years. I'm starting to feel tired of the moves and the hassle and stress that comes with each one. Age takes its toll, and I'm still young, but I definitely started feeling the need to simplify more, have fewer things, or stop moving.

I was really expecting a white Christmas; after all, it was one of those movie moments that was expected up north. With the scooter money, we bought ourselves skis and ski boots and were really looking forward to enjoying the one good thing about freezing for the next four months: *skiing*. We looked online at all the ski places we could get to by car, as traveling was expensive. A cab or Uber to the airport was an average of $120 one way, which meant that every time we wanted to fly, we needed to spend at least $240—and we hadn't even boarded the airplane. Traveling by car would be our only option. We booked a ski vacation in Montreal, Canada, for Simon's birthday (December 31), and we reserved the hotel with points.

It was close to Christmas, and no snow had fallen. I was surprised at how dark the streets were in the area. There were no street lights at all. We saw people taking their dogs for a walk with flashlights on their heads; otherwise, they couldn't even walk out without stumbling. It was pitch black. It was already getting dark early at night, and I felt isolated most of the day. When Simon arrived from work, I was like a dog. As soon as I saw the car arrive in the driveway, I rushed to the door and wagged my tail! Simon is home! Simon is home! I looked forward to his arrival all day I was becoming *Desperate Housewives of Norwalk*.

On the weekends, he took me on a "doggy" ride. As I can't drive at night due to my vision, and, with little daylight, I was dependent on Simon to take me out.

I started writing Christmas cards to send to friends and family in the United States and abroad and I saw a side effect I hadn't noticed before. My spelling was *awful*! I didn't know how to write the simplest of words. Every time I had written before, my spelling was corrected by autocorrect on the phone or computer. But when I tried to write things by hand, I couldn't spell *yesterday*, or *beautiful*. Nothing in any of my three languages. This was amazing and shocking. It's still the same. No change; no progress. I had good grammar, but now, it's pathetic.

For Christmas 2015, life's gift was not snow but the greatest gift of all, one that was about to change our lives completely and forever—a *baby*! I was pregnant! I found out a week before Christmas. We were not trying per se, but we had opened the possibility of having a baby by stopping the pills a couple of months ago. We thought it would take several months as I had been taking the pill for years plus all the medications I had to take after the surgery. So we really didn't expect it to happen so quickly. I couldn't believe the little blue plus sign on the pregnancy test, so I did two more. When all three tests gave me the same result, I was so happy that I immediately searched for a Babies "R" Us store to buy something to give Simon the news in a special way. I bought two baby socks, one pink and one blue with white polka dots and a little gift bag.

I drove home and waited patiently for Simon to arrive. If it normally felt like forever waiting for him to arrive, it felt even longer that day. On top of that, he worked later than usual. I was looking forward to sharing the news with him. Finally, he arrived home and I told him to sit on the sofa. I put my arms behind my back and asked him to pick a hand. He picked, and I gave him something gift wrapped. He unwrapped it, and it was the two little socks. He didn't understood for a few seconds. When he finally realized what it meant, he burst into tears of happiness. It was adorable to see him so happy! Of course, I was as well.

I gave him then the second package, which was the small gift bag containing the three pregnancy tests. I said, "Just in case there is any doubt, I took three tests."

Simon celebrated with a Johnnie Walker Blue Label drink that night, and me with water, now that I knew my drinking pleasure had ended for the next nine months. We called our parents to share the news with them and the next day, my sisters. I also couldn't wait to tell Elena, one of my best friends from Colombia, as she had told me she was pregnant with her first child only two weeks before. Since that moment, we have had the lucky pleasure of sharing our pregnancy adventures.

We hung the little socks on the Christmas tree and will have them there for all the Christmases to come.

But wait! Now I was pregnant, but we had already planned our ski trip and bought all the ski equipment. I rushed to get an appointment with the OB/GYN to ask if I could ski or not. He said that as long as I take it easy and ski at a significantly lower level than I normally do, it was fine. So we ended up going to ski, but I couldn't enjoy most of the pleasures of the trip. Après-ski? No drinking. Fondue? No unpasteurized cheese. Jacuzzi? No can-do while pregnant. Skiing nonstop from the first run until closing time? I didn't have the energy, nor could risk it. So I skied a maximum two or three hours a day.

Mount Tremblant was pretty, typical Canadian ski village. There was barely any snow on the first day, then we had a storm so we couldn't ski. We finally enjoyed the last day, but the slopes were so crowded, it was not a pleasure at all! We did one run and then had to queue up for an hour just to get the next lift. In addition, most of the slopes were closed, so the queues were insane. It was definitely far from the best skiing trip, but it was better than nothing, and, hey, I was pregnant! It would probably be one of the last trips for some time. So we had to enjoy it with its advantages and disadvantages.

We had spent Simon's birthday, New Year's, at the W in Montreal. It's a lovely city and is very romantic in the winter with its cute little French-style restaurants and neighborhoods. If only I could eat oysters and foie gras and drink champagne…oh well. You especially miss these things once you are forbidden to eat them. We headed back to Norwalk and started the new routine in our new lives.

Winter was tough. I didn't think it would be so hard. I was happy thinking about becoming a mother, but my days were lonely. Simon was at work all day long and it was impossible to meet people. In winter, people spend their time inside their houses, like we did. It was dark all the time and so cold that we didn't want to go out at all. I continued to go to the gym, but once the nausea from the pregnancy kicked in, I lost the motivation. Since then, I haven't been able to pick it up again. I know it's important for health and pregnancy, but I haven't been able to restart.

Now that I was back from vacation and installed in the house, my priority was to restart my therapies. I had never imagined how difficult this would be for me in this part of the United States. It took forever. There were long waiting lists and no doctor or therapy would take me without a referral, even though my insurance didn't require them. So first I had to get a general doctor (which could take three weeks for the first visit) to get the referral for a neurologist (which would take a month or more to get the appointment), who then had to refer me to a neuropsychologist and cognitive therapy (which would then take two months of waiting) and neurosurgeon.

With this long process, my first neuropsychology appointment was in April, and therapy would start four weeks later. This meant I had four months of waiting, but I wasn't going to sit around and do nothing! I continued doing the therapies I did in Miami with the four brain apps I have, which do pretty much the same exercises I did in the neuropsychologist office in Miami and continued with the cognitive-therapy book I was given. Those therapies were becoming boring, so I created new therapies for myself.

I discovered that MIT has published dozens of free classes online. So I started taking classes like the ones I had in college, thinking they could be good therapies. I connected the TV to the Internet and played the different classes on probability, statistics, quantum physics, micro and macroeconomics, and so on. I found everything interesting. I listened, took notes, and then tried to do the "homework" associated with them. It was strange, as when the concepts and definitions were explained, I knew everything I had done before in college, but when I tried to do the exercises, I couldn't. My brain couldn't. I continued trying but failed nonstop. If I could barely divide, how could I do integrals…oh well. I had to try. And try I did, but I failed.

I tried doing simpler tasks, like cooking. Being bad at

cooking I thought, *Great—some time to learn, and it must be a good exercise of coordination and remembering ingredients*. I bought all the cooking equipment and started trying. I failed, big time. Everything tasted like shit! I followed recipes to the letter, but nothing. On top of that, it took me forever, as with my short-term memory, I read an instruction and then forgot it. I had to read it again and again to once more forget it. I looked like a rat in a maze, completely lost. I felt bad about how much food I threw away because nothing tasted good. After a month of trying, my nausea was really bad and I couldn't stand any smells, so cooking was out of the question. The only thing I managed was banana bread, which Simon loves. Oh well, at least one success to put on the books.

What else could I do for new therapies? What about writing a book? It would help with my spelling, organizing the ideas in my head, short-term memory as I would need to remember what I wrote, and in overall exercising my brain! It must be good therapy.

So I started writing this book. I didn't know, and I still don't know, if it will be a good book or a shitty one, but it is my book. My first priority is writing as a form of therapy. In addition, I thought that when my baby is grown up, she won't ever know how I was prior to my surgery or the experience I've had with it, because by the time she can read, write, and understand I will have probably forgotten many details. So I would love to share my life with her. So this book is also for her and, if I have more children, for them.

When I started reading books from other patients, I couldn't find many out there. So I thought that maybe, like me, there are other patients who are looking to read about the experience of other patients and general life lessons. Maybe I could help others by writing about my experience. These are the reasons for *8-Rediscovering Life After a Brain Tumor*.

There was barely any snow that year and winter really hit me hard. I didn't realize how much until we took a trip to my father's apartment in Palm Beach for a week's vacation. We had a lovely time there, but it was hard because we realized how much we missed Miami, our friends, our house, the weather, and the things we liked to do. We drove past our now-rented house and I could not stop my tears. I felt so bad because Simon felt guilty for taking me to Norwalk. But this was not his fault at all! We had agreed together and made a rational decision together. Unfortunately, being in Miami made us realize we missed it a lot. I really didn't want to go back to the lonely life I was living. The cold weather, the dark days. We had lived there for four months. I still didn't know a single person other than Simon and he had not made any friends at work. Nani threw us a lovely surprise baby shower, which made us so happy! It also made me realize how lonely I was up north. In Miami, I also saw my dad and Antonella easily, as they traveled to Palm Beach and to visit us, but in the north, we didn't have many visits. My mom came by once, but that was it for a year.

March 31, 2016 was a day to remember, not only because it was my father's birthday and we were spending it together in Palm Beach, but because I received a wonderful call. While my dad wandered off to Target and Simon was working back in the apartment, I received a call from Reliance Standard, my disability-insurance carrier.

Finally, I received a call. I was approved for my long-term disability! I shouted in happiness, and tears fell down my cheeks in the middle of Target. I was disabled. Hurray! Yes, I was sad to be disabled, but I was happy as economically it was a help, and Simon and I needed that good news. Antonella was beside me at that moment and we both shouted and started jumping up and down in happiness. I had mixed feelings, but the predominant one was relief.

The person who called explained that it was approved for a year or so my file would be reviewed again as they would only continue approval if, by that time, I was "totally disabled." That day, I only wanted to celebrate and enjoy that one short call and my dad's birthday. I immediately called Simon, and we finished a happy day with dinner for my dad's birthday, some champagne to celebrate the disability, and sparkling water for me. And, if the day could not go better, it did! Simon and I had our hands on my belly when we suddenly felt the baby move for the first time. What a wonderful day! What a happy March 31st this was.

We travelled back to Norwalk. Arriving at the house was so hard for me. I was again in my prison of loneliness during the day. It was cold, snowy, and dark. Not being able to work, not being able to have any activities, not doing anything other than therapy was not fun at all. It was a tough moment. I tried seeing a psychologist so that I could vent at least, but there were none in the area with my insurance, and a private one would be too expensive. I asked if the one I was seeing in Miami would take my appointments via Skype, but he explained that he could not bill the insurance unless my home address was still in Florida. This option didn't work out.

Now that the insurance had kicked in and I was soon to receive my first disability check, I could not stop thinking, *if only we had known of this approval in time, we wouldn't have had to change our lives completely and move up here.* We could have afforded our house at least while the disability was there and continued with my therapies, my friends, and my pregnancy in our house that we loved so much. I was pissed off. Why did they take so long? Didn't they have any sense of how much the time they take to make a decision can affect another person's life emotionally and economically? We wouldn't have to be in this lonely, boring little town, where my only company during the day were the people I called on the phone or Skype. Damn it! I missed Miami and now we knew we could have stayed there.

It was too late now. We were there, in what I call "the

freezer." There was no turning back. I had to accept it. I was still grateful to be approved for the disability, but if only it would have happened at a more appropriate time.

Maybe a dog would be great company for me. I looked at breeders of my favorite breed, which are Samoyeds, got the price, and bought a book on how to train them as I have never had a dog before. I read it completely, watched many videos online about how to train them, and was about to reserve and pay for it. I had even picked the name. The added value was that my peripheral eyesight was not back, so I could train it as a guide dog to help me out. It was a done deal...except when I started reading and asking a bit more about having a puppy and a baby at the same time. I found many incidents of the puppy not accepting or liking the baby and families had to give the dog away. It seems that this doesn't happen when the dog is older, but, in my case, the puppy would still be a puppy by the time the baby was born. So we decided to postpone getting the dog.

Oh well, that was that. I needed to look for another type of company. Intensive Skype would again be the solution.

I started to notice my brain fatigue more and more as I tried to do things. When I added more activities to my agenda, I really noticed it. For example, one time I was invited to the Hamptons for a weekend (Saturday to Sunday) with a friend from my MBA. I had such a lovely time with them and Simon. We went right after a lot of snow had fallen, and it was gorgeous to see snow on the beach! We had a nice relaxing weekend of chatting, fire time, eating, and walking along the beach. The first day I felt normal. The following day, boom! That's when the brain fatigue kicked in. I hadn't realized how much of a toll keeping up with conversations with people for more than a couple of hours would take on me the next day. I couldn't even speak in the car on the way home. It took me three or four days to recover as I was brain-dead.

I started looking at volunteer work since I had some free time, I would love to help people out if I could. In our busy lives, it is difficult to find time to help out, but I had all the time in the world now, except the time I needed to dedicate to therapy and recharging my batteries. I looked online and applied to different places. After sending many documents and background checks, I got into three volunteering jobs. The first one I started was a program with the Connecticut government for the legally blind. I started visiting and helping one person out once a week at his home. He was a lovely Russian man who had lost his wife a year ago. He was capable of doing most of the things by himself, but he was quite lonely, so my weekly visits made him happy. They made me happy too. Helping someone gave me joy.

Around the same time, I also started reading books to young children who had difficulty reading. I was especially looking forward to having this experience as I had never really been close to children. In my family, I didn't have nearby children. There was only one, my nephew, but he lived in a different country from me, so I didn't share much with him.

Children are great. They're so innocent, sweet and grateful. The things they say are adorable and unexpected. I had two children, each for thirty minutes. The girl was always dressed up with the cutest of clothes. A yellow tutu was her favorite. She loved reading long books and made great voices and sang along with the book. The little boy was a slow reader and had a very short attention span. He liked *I Spy*, and it was difficult to convince him to try different books. Both were African American children.

After some time, they started sharing a bit of their personal lives with me. The little girl was admirable. She lived with her mother and both sets of grandparents in the same house. On the weekends, she took care of all of them as they had health issues, including helping to bathe them. She described what she did with love and she was happy about being able to help them. How different lives can be.

The third volunteering job I found was at the Connecticut Brain Tumor Society. They were organizing a golf tournament to raise funds and I helped them out with a bit of Excel, adding information into it. It was a minor amount of help for all the work they did, but I couldn't do much more as I already had the two other volunteer jobs plus my therapy and my doctors' appointments (which, with the pregnancy, started multiplying). This alone was a therapy and this simple task that once would of taken me 30 minutes, took several days to complete.

I worked from a distance with two people who have been so special to me since we first spoke. Kimberly, especially, has been special and understanding. I still haven't met her in person, but every time we have spoken over the phone, she was so supportive and caring. What a special person! I didn't get the chance to go to the tournament, as it was a long drive. Once the golf tournament was over, she helped me by reading my book and editing it. I am immensely grateful, as I didn't know anyone in the industry.

But oh my, how much we missed Miami and our house. It was amazing how much we missed our lives there. We never missed Puerto Rico like this, and I had never missed anywhere else once I had moved. I would always move on. I had the strange feeling of missing Miami, and still do. I needed to stop missing it. I needed to move on. What was wrong with me? I am a strong, rational person. Why was I still stuck on this? I truly didn't understand. Maybe someone could help me understand. Being simpleminded was easier. Not being able to process thoughts and just enjoying coloring had given me so much happiness.

I needed to find a way to grasp those moments. Happiness can be simple, and it's actually easier when it's simpler. I had to stop these thoughts from coming to my brain. I had nothing to complain about; life was perfect. I had perfect husband who supported me, a new place, a new experience—shitty weather, yes, but with a nice cozy fireplace. Stop it, Nathalie! Be happy.

Dad and Antonella helped me with Tata, a great psychologist in Colombia who agreed to see me via Skype. I've been speaking to her for some months now. She has been a great support. She not only listens but is also practical and gives me advice, and we work together on plans so that I can not only cope and mentally start organizing a future for myself but also help me see that there are new paths I can take in my life. I told her about the book I was writing and she generously offered to read it and give me her feedback, which I'm so thankful for. I know she will continue to be a great support.

Finally, it was time for my famous, long-awaited neurologist's appointment at Gaylord Hospital and the neurosurgeon. At Yale, I met with Andrea, not the neurosurgeon. The purpose was to touch base and get things prepared for when I could actually have a new MRI after giving birth. We spent more than an hour together. She was the nicest, most caring head nurse I had ever met. She was extremely nice and understanding. She showed me around the hospital and took me to the volunteering office if I wanted to try to volunteer there as well. She even accompanied me to the parking lot twice, as I had forgotten to stamp the parking ticket. When have you had anyone from the medical office accompany you to the parking lot as a nice gesture? I would guess never. She had also had a brain tumor removed some time ago, though her side effects were different. We had that in common, but, nevertheless, we got along so well. It's strange how much emotional impact one person can have on you. I have never felt so grateful to anyone in the medical field. It was one extremely kind gesture, and I will never forget her.

The following day, I had the neuropsychology test done. It was a long day of testing. I arrived at nine in the morning and finished at four. I would get the results in two weeks. I was looking forward to seeing the progress I had made in the seven months since the last testing. After so many hours of therapy, both in therapy sessions and on my own for hours at home, reading books, and free online MIT classes, and so on, I was certain there would be so much improvement. Was I back to normal? I didn't feel like that, but maybe I was and I was being too hard on myself. After the test I was completely out of it. I probably shouldn't have driven back, my brain was fatigued and to make matters worse, there was torrential rain.

I knew the brain fatigue was still hard on me, and my vision had not come back, but IQ-wise, I had my hopes up. Would I soon be able to go back to work? Or if not soon, for sure after the baby was born? I noticed with no doubt that my math was still completely off and simple division was still impossible. Noticing this, I thought I could find a career with less numbers, like law. I researched online, and Yale, being close by, could be an option. I downloaded the LSAT mock questions to see how well I could do on this. Maybe I could become a lawyer? I planned to take this question to the neurophysiologist once I saw my results. Again, plan A was normal, and plan B was normal with fewer numbers. That sounded like a wise plan.

After more than a year after my surgery (my "craniversary," anniversary of my craniotomy), I was finally going to get the "you are back to normal" news! I was already thinking how to celebrate. There weren't many options, as I couldn't ski now that I was further into my pregnancy. Zika virus had become a World Health Organization threat for pregnant women, so traveling to the tropics and the Caribbean Islands was not an option. I would find another way to celebrate, no worries. That would be easy to find. A couple of days before the appointment for the results, the neuropsychologist called me and asked me to please come in with Simon. Mmm…that was strange. Why did I need to come in with him? Did this mean she didn't have good news? Maybe taking another person was just part of the procedure? I would need to wait anyway, so we waited, and Simon made an opening in his work agenda to accompany me. The journey took one hour but felt like three. I was very nervous, put on my stubborn brave face.

"Based on her background history, high average and above premorbid intellectual abilities are estimated. At this time, her current intellectual skills were found to be in the *low average* range. Overall, given her estimated premorbid intellectual abilities and the results of previous testing obtained in July 18, 2014, an overall decline in intellectual function was found twelve months' post-resection,"[11] said the neuropsychologist.

"Your FSIQ is 89, low average range", she said.

I kind of stopped listening, even though the appointment went on for a complete hour where she did not stop talking and explaining the detailed results and findings of the test and conclusions. I didn't stop listening because of a lack of interest; I was going into shock when in more normal, nonmedical words, she said, "There are basically no improvements in the six months since your last test.".

What! *No* improvements? None at all? Nothing? How could that be? After all those hours, days, weeks and months of therapy? After all the effort I made? None? No! No, no, no. Impossible. No!

Before the surgery my IQ was 114 (in my second language), and now 89! If there had not been any improvements at all in the past seven months, how could there be any additional in the future?

---

[11] Neuropsychologist testing results, 2016.

Shit! Below average was my new brain forever? No. Impossible.

She explained that most of the recovery happens in the first six months to a year. Once we passed that mark of twelve months post-surgery, the tipping point happens in terms of how much the brain can recover. Most (over 90 percent) is expected to recover. Yes, there can be a bit more recovery, but the biggest improvements had been made. So if there had not been many improvements in the last seven months, even though some could still happen, they would be significantly smaller improvements. That meant this was basically it in terms of my improvements.

She stated that I was still disabled. She also recommended that in order to manage my brain fatigue, I needed to space out my activities. So if I did things one day, the next day I had to make sure to not do anything in order to recharge my batteries. It would be the only way to manage the fatigue, learning how to cope with it, as this side effect would be permanent.

Knowing the baby was coming, she recommended making sure I had people to help, as coping with brain fatigue combined with sleepless nights is not a good recipe. She said she would do the next test in twelve months' time to see if there were any improvements and told me to continue doing therapy, hoping maybe more improvements could happen. She also recommends focusing on only one task at a time, and to not do anymore multitasking. My brain wouldn't manage it and I would only forget things. I needed to write everything down in order to not forget things. Always put things in the same spot, so I knew how to retrieve them. Take breaks when needed in order to avoid cognitive fatigue.

I asked her, "So this is not only about numbers? Because I had thought that maybe I could, for example, study law, if the numbers were the part of the brain that was not really working out."

She explained that, unfortunately, my cognitive deficits went above and beyond only numbers. Law or any "higher thinking" requires analysis of factors and variables, finding solutions to problems, and being able to see options. My brain was so simple that it was not capable of seeing different paths to the same solution, therefore I got stuck on one option and was not capable of figuring out different options. In addition to that, learning anything new would be highly difficult because of my lack of short term memory. So a new career, independent of what it was, would be extremely challenging with no short-term memory for new things. Before the surgery, Simon had bought Rosetta Stone in Italian, and I had been learning that fourth language for a couple of months. I thought this free time was perfect for this too. Now that sounded like an impossible task. I could try, but how many years would I need to dedicate to it if I forget every new thing I learned?

I arrived home and I was in so much shock that I didn't cry. I didn't want to accept this. I didn't even call my parents. I didn't tell anyone. I didn't want to speak. Simon asked me several times how I was, what was I feeling, but I just didn't want to speak. I was in denial. My family called me several times to ask me how the appointment went, as they knew I was going, but I didn't answer the phone. I didn't want to speak.

I went to bed, turned on the TV and wanted the world to suck me in and make me disappear. I didn't speak to anyone for two days, until I finally cried alone in the house and then to Simon when he arrived home. Oh boy, did I cry this time. This was it. This was the end of the recovery path. I knew that. This was the moment where hopes had been destroyed. I needed to accept my new self as soon as I had absorbed the shock. It was the end of the road—this particular road.

How unlucky could I be? How was it possible that I got all the worst side effects, and they were here for life? How was it possible that I wouldn't be able to go back to the work I loved? I signed on for a simple, short surgery, with only a small chance of losing my peripheral eyesight, and one year later, I was facing major cognitive and visual deficits for life?

Please don't let my ability to work and make my own living be taken away! How would I ever be able to maintain myself in the future? Yes, Simon was with me, but what if he wasn't at some point in the future? Would I be helpless forever? What about my baby? How was I supposed to care for her and offer her everything she deserved if I can't work? I felt defenseless and powerless, a victim of no one but my brain. Simon, the love of my life would help me and our baby and would always be there for me, but life is so long, and so many things can happen. I couldn't take it for granted. No one can or should.

Big changes needed to happen. We needed to sell the house. Even if the disability was approved, the house was still over our budget in the longer term with only one salary. We were building dreams together and now we had to sell everything we put so much into.

I was still incapable of saying the findings of the testing out loud. I asked Simon to call my parents and tell them, because I didn't want to hear those words come out of my mouth. To date, I haven't told anyone, not even my sisters. Anyone who reads this will probably find out for the first time.

I didn't want to accept this or admit it. I wasn't ready. I had so much to look forward, and I would soon be a mother, but I needed to process the feelings. I needed to grieve for my brain or for the loss of it before I could be fully emotionally prepared to let go of the bad news and to turn the page, a new chapter, filled with joy, love, and happiness.

But I still needed to process the news. I had to accept my new reality. Even if my brain did get better and I could do other types of work, my brain fatigue wouldn't allow me to work a full-time, five-day week. I had to accept that I would never be able to work, even in a simple job. So Simon and I needed to manage a new way of life. I was sure it would be a happy one, but we needed to make significant adjustments.

I felt so bad for Simon. This was so unfair to him. He worked hard all his life. So had I. But he came from a life with fewer luxuries than I had and now that he had arrived in a place where he could enjoy hobbies and things he deserves like golf, traveling, concerts, restaurants, and so on, I became an economical burden on him, and we had to strongly limit how we lived in order to pay the bills and save for our baby. It was so unfair. He generously insisted that it didn't affect him, that he was happy to maintain me and his new family, but I still think it had to be difficult for him, as we didn't have enough for him to do even some of his hobbies. I had the brain tumor, but he has to pay for the consequences too. I'm so sorry. I'm grateful, but so sorry I had become a burden for him when before I was the breadwinner. I felt sorry for myself too.

If only I had known the risks of the surgery and its effects, I would have made completely different decisions. Maybe I wouldn't have had the surgery at all, although the doctor did recommend it as the tumor could have continued growing, but who knows what permanent effects. Fine, the surgery was needed, but was it needed so quickly? I could have waited six months and, in that time, prepared for these types of consequences. I could have bought better life insurance or better disability insurance. I could have worked until the yearly bonus was paid. It was important money, especially when there was a possibility of never being able to work again.

I felt mad that I didn't know more information before the surgery. Why were we given such a light, positive outlook? Why didn't the doctor and nurse give us a broader perspective of what could go wrong? Why were we not given more information to prepare ourselves? They could at least have been more negative, so we would understand the complexity of the situation and acted upon it more significantly. Maybe if I had known all these risks, I would have been so scared I wouldn't have gone into surgery. If I had known all these possible side effects, instead of laughing away being so dumb, I might have fallen into a deep depression when I got all these side effects immediately after surgery.

I will never know, will I? It is what it is. The side effects are what they are. My new reality is what it is now. My future? I don't know what it will be. Normally we have a path in life that we work for, study for, hope for, plan for. I don't anymore. I have my education and my memories but no longer my abilities. I have a blank page. A completely white page, with only four words written on it: *Simon* and *my baby*.

CHAPTER EIGHT

BRAIN TUMOR STILL HAUNTING ME?

I thought I was finished writing the book. I also thought after Nicole's birth, my mind and feelings regarding my surgery automatically would have been forgotten and a real new book of my life would start. Little I knew the brain tumor would continue to haunt me for a little while longer.

August 15, 2016 at 12.01 a.m. my water breaks. My contractions were still a part so we waited, but 30 minutes later, they started to get closer together. So we got on our way to the hospital. Yes, the big moment! We were now really close to meeting our little Nicole. Once we arrived at the hospital, the MD checked me, but I wasn't dilated enough, so they made me walk the corridors. I find myself walking through hospitals corridors again. A completely different reason for this walk. It was so painful! Everyone says its painful, but I would have never imagined it could possibly feel worse than it was at that moment. Until 5 hours later, I felt I was going to have a heart attack from the pain! On my god! This was PAIN! The nurse definitely saw the difference in the pain level, so she put in the epidural. The epidural made its effect, I had no more pain, but it slowed contractions down. I started pushing at 6:00a.m. The baby only came out by 6:00p.m.

The first time I saw my baby I couldn't stop crying of happiness. It is amazing how strong the maternal instinct is. It kicked in like a huge wave into my heart! I was feeling an uncontrollable, gigantic, extreme love. Like I had never felt before. All those doubts I had about being or not a mother completely vanished in a millisecond. I was overwhelmed with love towards my little Nicole. I was so happy! I was so in love. The nurse brought her to my chest and there she was. My little baby. Nothing would ever separate us.

After breastfeeding or at least trying -it's not easy at the beginning when it's your first time and all those baby books I read before weren't helping much at that moment, I had not eaten or slept now in a day, physically destroyed, exhausted after pushing - I had the strongest and worst brain fatigue ever. I needed to sleep and recover. Of course I couldn't sleep though. My baby now needed to eat every 2 hours. But I was so tired! So tired! So physically broken and torn, my brain was barely functioning. All moms go through this, but with my brain fatigue, I felt my exhaustion to another level. I could barely speak. I was stuttering again. A lot. I just needed a rest to be ok again. But that rest would not come to me in months.

As I had a vaginal delivery, I would be allowed to stay in the hospital 2 nights. We asked our OBGYN if it would be possible to stay a third night due to my brain fatigue, so in order to do this she asked the hospital's neurologist to come and see me. He came, asked me some brief questions. Simon and I explained about my craniotomy in 2015. He did write the note to my OBGYN, so they allowed us to stay one more night. He could clearly see I was brain fatigued. The days passed quick. The neurologist recommended I have my routine brain MRI done in the hospital, as being an in-patient at the hospital would be easier than being an out-patient. So we left Nicole at the hospital's nursery, Simon went home to sort things there for my arrival and go food shopping. The MRI takes usually one hour, so we planned it in between feeds.

When I came back to my room, I called the nurse via the in-room voice-call service and asked them to bring me back Nicole as it was time to feed her.

"We can't take Nicole back to you", the nurse replied.

Wait, what? What? What do you mean "you can't bring my baby to me?". It was feeding time! She was hungry. I demanded they bring me back my daughter. So the nurse came in to my room and said:

"I cannot bring Nicole to you. You cannot be left alone with your daughter. It is an order from the Social Worker".

"What do you mean the social worker? The one that came yesterday and saw me for a short period of time?" I replied.

"Yes. That one. She gave the order that you cannot be left alone or unsupervised with your daughter from now until she turns one year old. Never unsupervised. The reason being your brain fatigue and your short-term memory".

"WHAT!? This is absolutely CRAZY! This is so wrong! I demand to speak with her. Bring her in please. NOW! I need to feed my baby!"

After seeing how mad I was, the nurse made an exception because it was time to feed Nicole, so she brought her in. She stayed with me to supervise. I called Simon immediately and told him the situation. He was off course, got as mad as I was. This is ridiculous! He came back to the hospital and demanded to see the social worker. They managed to find her and she came to the room. She explained that because I had a brain surgery and had a short term memory issues she already signed the order that I can't be left alone with Nicole for the first year of her life. If I ever did, social workers would have the right to take her away from me. She said it was to protect the baby. It was for her own good. Simon and I explained that my short term memory is for numbers, for names. Not at all for forgetting I had a baby! She did not care and said, she would not change her verdict.

Simon and I were so mad. So upset. So pissed off. A completely wrong verdict from a social worker that saw me five minutes the prior day and did not even ask about what type of brain tumor I had, or what were the side effects of it. A person that took an ignorant decision that would affect the rest of my year. My first year with Nicole. A decision that instead of helping would make my life impossible. Impossible! I have no family here. How I am supposed to never be left alone with my daughter? So when Simon is working, what do I do? When Simon goes food shopping, what do I do? The social worker responded to that: "well get a neighbor to come and supervise you. Or you go and do the food shopping and leave Nicole with the father". Get a babysitter, what for a year? What about when Simon would need to travel? I can't afford a day time sitter, even less a night time sitter. This was a real problem. There it was. My brain tumor again returning to haunt me. How can a brain tumor affect me this way! It was so unfair. I felt like a piece of my heart had been broken by that social worker by separating me from my daughter. She had taken away the right of a mother to be with her daughter the first year of her life.

Time to leave the hospital. We leave with our little Nicole. We arrive home to that first night that terrifies all new parents. Of course in the hospital you know you have help and a lot of people with expertise on the matter. Two parents alone with a new born is scary! And of course, that first night was a nightmare. She cried all day and night. We didn't understand what was happening, so we took her to the pediatrician. They explained I was probably not making enough milk, so we had to supplement. She was crying nonstop as she was simply hungry.

Leaving the house was so difficult. I was still in so much pain. So the first week in the house with Simon, instead of enjoying the moment, enjoying our new little princess and recovering physically, I had to focus all my energy (the little energy I had with sleepless nights) to call all my doctors and get appointments to get them to document and write letters to debunk the decision the social worker had done. In between of my pain, the lack of sleep and my hormones all over the place, every single call I made I could not stop crying when I would explain to the doctors schedulers, that I needed an emergency appointment with them. I called my neurologist, my neurosurgeon, my OBGYN, my neuropsychologist and my speech therapist. Got appointments with all of them.

In the meantime a Plan B had to be put in place. What if I still had the ban when Simon had to return to work, which was one month after his paternity leave. My father helped me by sending to me our grandmothers maid, Rosita, from Colombia to help me out in the house for 3 months. She would arrive one month after Nicole's birth, exactly when Simon would go back to work. This way, I would not "be left alone with the baby".

The second week was so difficult. I was still in pain, and now I would have to drive and go to medical appointments to get the letters. I felt so mad. I should be enjoying this moment and this woman has made it a nightmare. When I managed to see all the doctors, they all had the same reaction.

"This is CRAZY, the social worker should have never done this to you."

They all wrote a letter explaining that it was absolutely OK for me to be left alone with my daughter. My short term memory challenge was a very different type of short term memory issue. Simon and I sent the letters to the OBGYN and by Nicole's first month, I was finally able to be left alone with her. I was finally a normal mom.

Being a new parent is the best thing ever. I never understood what everybody fussed about so much when they said, "being a parent is the best thing that can happen to anyone". I finally understood. What a strong feeling, surreal. Inexplicable. The most powerful feeling ever. It physically and emotionally rewires you. Suddenly I love not only my baby, but all babies. This feeling of love also comes with tears, every time I see in the news that someone's child got murdered or dies I can't stop crying. I find it fascinating how nature changes you and your instincts.

After we had solved this problem, we decided that we needed to downsize. We made a mistake when calculating the amount we could afford in rent, as we didn't take into account the high costs of heating, snow clearing and gardening. We were still waiting for the court date for Social Security disability case and did not know the outcome of the trial. So we had to move again. Having Rosita with us would be an extra pair of hands for the move, so definitely better to move while she was with us, than after she had gone back to Colombia. We found a very nice apartment building in Norwalk called the Quincy Lofts, with 1 and 2 bedroom apartments. The landlords in addition wanted to increase our rent after only one year with them, so we decided it was time to move.

I had never imagined how much the move would change my life in Connecticut. It was full of positive surprises. First, living in a smaller apartment, one open space made it so much easier with Nicole. Laundry, kitchen, living room and dining room in the same space. I could watch over Nicole with ought going up and down the stairs. Making life easier with a newborn is so important. Rosita left two weeks after we were in the apartment. By coincidence, one week after I moved into the apartment, my next door neighbor did too. She also had daughter a little bit older than Nicole. She was so sweet. I invited her over, and we got well immediately! She changed my life here. I finally had a friend! My first Connecticut friend. I told her about my book, and she read it in one day. That was so sweet of her. That really touched me. Winter arrived and we would spend hours in our apartments, just chatting, laughing, playing with our daughters. Walking down the corridor towards the elevator on my same floor, I saw another mom with a stroller. As I had such a good experience with Alyssa, I decided to talk to her and ask if she wanted to come over to my apartment. That's how I met my second Connecticut friend Tanya and Kaiden, Nicole's first baby friend. From no friends in CT, to two! Another day in the lobby, another mom with a newborn was there. I approached her to get together as well and we become close friends too! Courtney became my third mom friend. It was starting to be so much fun to have mom friends. They filled my days and my little Nicole's with joy. I kind of liked it and felt again the little social bee I used to be back in college and MBA. I created a little mom community of like 10 moms in the building. With a "Whatsapp" group to chat amongst us, go to happy hours, playdates and meet in our apartments or playgrounds. I was having so much fun being a mom. My little Nicole just lights my eyes up and in addition finally some friends! Life was starting to get sweeter. Finally. After years of a rough run.

When I was having fun with my friends and Nicole, I wouldn't think of the surgery nor the side effects. But in my quiet moments, I could not avoid going back to my memories. Going back to thinking, who am I now? Yes I'm a mom, a stay at home mom now, but who am I? Who am I if I don't work? If as an individual I'm no one. I felt useful when I was volunteering, but now that I don't have the time with Nicole, nor the money for a sitter, am I only a mom? I want to continue helping people. I want to find a way with my new schedule.

During my recovery, I found a lot of support through online Facebook brain tumor survivor groups in the USA. It's a safe place to share your feelings, vent, ask questions and listen to other patients stories. A safe place to share thoughts you might not want to share with your family or husband. Feelings of fear, of doubt, pain or sadness. Feelings you might think they don't understand, but other fellow survivors might. I also started to go to YALE for the brain tumor survivor groups. These groups gave me strength. I drove once a week to meet them at the Smillow Cancer Center. It was the first time I met real brain tumor survivor patients, and not only online. It was so special to me. Andrea Laudano, which I had mentioned before was always there and would be so kind to me and my little Nicole. Nicole was so cute and would just crawl all over the room and in a way lighten an otherwise sad room. Hearing other patients stories, specially fellow patients that actually had terminal brain tumors, made me realize I had nothing to complain about. Nothing at all. I should not feel any pity for myself or feel sorry for myself. Not unlucky. Not unhealthy. The contrary. Shame on me, for feeling anything other than grateful! Grateful than I am alive. Grateful that my life was never in real risk. Lucky I never had a timer on it. At least, not an obvious one. Yes, yes with a lot of disabling deficits. Dumb and partially blind, but still had a long life ahead of me with my husband and daughter. I need to change my mindset. I need to be happy again! I need to be thankful. I need to start embracing a new life. A happy one. One that leaves the past behind and uses the learnings to make me a better human being. Not a smarter one, but a better one. Someone to feel proud off not because of my work career, but because of the person I have become. A strong, kind person that has overcome a brain tumor, not to help herself, but to help others. Yes! That has to be my new calling. Help others. I want this to be my new purpose in life. Be a great mom and help others.

When I realized how much Facebook groups helped me, I noticed some patients where posting in Spanish and not many people responded. That got me thinking, are there no groups for survivors in Latin America? So I looked them up and there were none. So I decided to create the first Facebook Group for brain tumor survivors in Latin America. It slowly started to grow and people from Spain started to join, which I thought was strange, but there wasn't any group in Spain either. I changed the name to include Spain to "Tumores Cerebrales España y Latinoamérica".

Finally the letter I had been waiting for months arrived! I had a court date for my Social Security Disability hearing on June 19, 2016 in New Haven. I had been waiting years for this to happen! I had applied on 2015. I called my disability lawyer, to make sure we had everything in place. She was still in Miami and social security does pay for your lawyer to travel for the hearing, so I kept the same one. When I managed to get a hold of her, she said unfortunately she could not make it to Connecticut, because she was pregnant and the month of my court date, was the same month of her giving birth. Shoot! What now? What was I going to do? I didn't want to change the court date because that would mean again waiting months, maybe years. I had already waited over two years for this date. I had to look for a new lawyer, but my trial was coming up in a couple of months. I had to now put all my energy and focus on finding a new lawyer. I called more than 10 firms, and no one would take my case because I already had a lawyer. I explained to them the situation and they simply did not even want to take a look at my file. I can't go with ought a lawyer to court. With my short term memory, my difficulty understanding, I would be lost in court. I probably would not even be able to explain myself well or not at all. So I continued calling and calling, until finally two people accepted to see me. The first a graduate from YALE. When I got there, after waiting for an hour, she said:

"Oh sorry. My assistant made a mistake. I had told her I

would not take your case. It is very difficult to prove totally disabled when it comes to brain disabilities. It is difficult to prove brain fatigue."

I had driven all the way to see her for her to say this? Now what! I only had one more option. I was so worried. So sad. I felt no one would support me or understand me. The following day I called Jeremy Virgil. After explaining my case to him, he immediately said he would take it! Finally I had hope. He just made my day! Possibly my future! I was so grateful! I took an appointment soon after that and went with my husband, little Nicole and all the paper work we had advanced with the previous lawyer. What an amazing lawyer he was. He was so kind, a great listener, understanding of our situation and understanding that we had our baby with us there. One hour after, he had all the details and paperwork needed for the case and he confirmed he could attend the court date. I would only need to meet him one more time before the hearing took place.

We met with Jeremy a couple of days before. His recommendation was to just be myself. The medical files should speak for themselves. Still, I was so nervous. What if I didn't understand or remember the questions I was asked? Could I trust my short term memory on this day? What if I had a lot of brain fatigue? He said not to worry, he was there to help and support me. I felt he had my back. Simon also had to come to testify if the judge wanted him to. Jeremy explained to me that court rooms are small. They are meant for us to feel comfortable, precisely as the people applying have disabilities. In addition to the judge, a disability examiner would be there to ask me questions.

The big day was here. Even if Jeremy had explained everything to me, I have never been to court. I wasn't 100% certain of what to expect. Other than what we see on TV, big court rooms with a lot of people sitting in them or the smaller owes like in the Judge Judy TV show. We went upstairs and looked for the waiting room. We spoke with a police officer in the entrance, before passing the metal detector. We waited for maybe 30-40 minutes before it was our turn. They called my name, and only mine. So Simon was not called in with me. I went in with Jeremy.

Inside the court room, it was much more intimidating than I thought! I had imagined a small room with normal tables. It was very intimidating because, even though it was a small room, the ALJ was sitting in a very real 'wooden judge stand' that was raised much higher than the level we were sitting. At our lower level, I sat down beside Jeremy. We both were facing the judge. To my right, a nice lady was typing everything we said. A guard that opened the door was standing behind. On the phone, dialed in on a conference number, was the disability examiner.

The judge said as soon as we came in and sat down:

"Raise your right hand. Do you solemn swear that you will tell the truth, the whole truth, and nothing but the truth, so help you god?

"Yes. I do. I swear.", I answered.

I didn't know which one of those to answer, so I answered with all the words that came into mind. I wasn't sure if I was raising my "right" hand. After my surgery I wasn't sure which was right and left. I was worried I could be offending the judge. So I started apologizing already and asking Jeremy if that was the correct side to raise my hand.

The administrative law judge asked me about my education, my background, what type of jobs I performed in the past, if have I had worked since I applied to SSD. He asked me about my disability conditions, doctors that have seen me. I explained the best I could. Jeremy kindly stepped in and asked me questions he thought I missed that were important for the judge to hear. I was so nervous I spoke in a quiet tone and the judge had to ask me several times to speak louder for him to hear. Once the judge finished asking questions, the person on the phone started stating that there were three types of jobs across the USA, for example I could work at a café. He stated the exact number of that exact type of job available in the country and in my state. That was where Jeremy stepped in and asked him, that with my short term memory, if I can't remember the correct orders of customers, would I be able to maintain that job? To which the answer was "no". I was given another example of a different job, but the answer was still that I could not maintain that job either. That intervention was so important from Jeremy. I would not have known what to answer or do if I had gone into court without him. Having a disability lawyer is key for anyone in this process. He was a total Rockstar! I admired him so much at that moment. After approximately 30 minutes in the courtroom, we had finished. The judge never called in Simon. Now we just had to wait. Wait for how long? More wait? He didn't give the verdict in the spot. Jeremy explained to me that it is normal for judge not to give us the verdict immediately. I would receive it in the mail in a couple of months. The wait continues.

In order to continue therapies with my little Nicole, I had to find a speech therapist closer to home, as with her I couldn't drive an hour back and forth every time to Gaylord. I found one across the street from the apartment building. She was very understanding and allowed me to take Nicole with me, as we couldn't afford a baby sitter. I went to sessions with her for approximately 6 more months in addition to all the years I had done previously with other therapies. After this time, she gave me a final evaluation and said she couldn't treat me anymore because I had plateaued. Insurance would not cover any more treatments as I couldn't progress anymore. I had arrived at the maximum I could get to in terms of recovery. This was the end of the recovery route. I had now to accept that the way I am, is the way I will be for the rest of my life. Knowing this last therapy, was the end of the recovery road gave me peace. I felt in peace because I had done over the years everything I possibly could to get better. I dedicated years to my recovery and went above and beyond I ever imagined doing (including writing this book). I also had started to notice it myself how I was not really improving anymore. I did everything I could to get better, and now it was time to do everything I can to create a new life with my little Nicole and Simon with new abilities and disabilities.

George, our USPS mailman, the best USPS mailman in the country, delivered to me the letter we were all waiting for! I was so nervous, and Simon wasn't home. I couldn't stop myself from opening the letter, so I did. I read it and didn't understand! So I ran to Alyssa's and rang the doorbell like crazy! I gave her the letter and asked her to explain to me what it said. Was I approved or not? It kind of said I was, but there were some legal jargon that made it confusing. She read it and told me yes! I was approved for social security disability! I couldn't stop jumping up and down! I was officially disabled! I felt so happy. I felt relieved, that a small economical help would be on the way. This was such an important help in our lives. I stopped one second to realize, I was disabled. For real. Oh my god, for real. So now I have tears in my eyes. I'm disabled. Legally disabled. I'm 36 years old and disabled. What a bitter sweet moment. I'm so happy, yet so sad. I smile and cry at the same time. Not many moments in one's life you can be on those two feelings at the same time triggered by one letter, the social security disability letter. I calmed down a bit, and just decided to enjoy the moment. That weekend we celebrated with Simon and of course my family over the phone.

The apartment we were renting, was very nice and practical, but it was starting to feel temporary, and not like home. Nicole was growing so quick we started thinking of her future growing up in a good school district and a house that would feel like home where she could run around, and have a backyard. So I started looking at Zillow hoping a smaller, more affordable home would come up for sale in Westport, New Canaan or Darien (as we had heard those three towns had much better schools than Norwalk). I looked every day, and with our realtor saw many houses, until we found one we loved! Almost the same size of the apartment, so still an easy to maintain size home with a Cape Cod architectural style. We made an offer a couple of days after seeing the house and moved in for Christmas.

The house surprisingly quickly felt like home. It felt like we had been living in it for years. As it was small, we didn't need furniture as we had everything already. The contrary, we actually had too much furniture, as the Miami house was bigger, so we had to get rid of the second sofa, and still haven't found place for the desk. The house has high vaulted ceilings in the chimney area. A great back yard terrace, cute rooms, good light and a great front porch. It needed some work though to not feel as old as it was. Built in 1928, it had the original uneven walls and ceilings, so we decided to make the home feel more modern inside. We put new sheetrock and evened out the walls. Painted them to our liking. Reclaimed the wooden floor, sanded it and painted it. The outside needed work too. We paved the road, painted the house as it hadn't been painted in years. We had to take three truckloads of leaves accumulated in the back yard that the previous owner never cleared out. Finally, after a lot of dust and work, the house was looking amazing! Home sweet home. The house had all the advantages of the apartment, easy to clean and maintain organized, easy to have on eye on Nicole every time as it was small, and still a home where I could invite friends and family over as now I had a guest bedroom. Love it! Compared to our home in Miami, it's different. Off course the pool in Miami was amazing, the house bigger, and more modern. Still, our new home had its own charm and I loved it. Simon did too. Nicole was starting to feel home as well.

The day we moved in, our next door neighbor very kindly came to present herself and invited us to an open house with friends and neighbors she was having the following week. So nice of her to welcome us to the neighborhood. Another big reason to feel like home so quick. The first week in, and I had met all my neighbors. They were all so nice and friendly. I got on well with all of them, but specially Hannah and Vincent, a very nice couple that had a toddler Nolan, the same age as Nicole. They had just bought their house in Westport but were moving in 2 months after we met. We exchanged phone numbers and I invited her over a couple of weeks after we met so that Nicole could meet Nolan. Our two toddlers being the same age, was ideal. We really got along well immediately and have become good friends. She moved in to her new home and we see each other almost every week ever since. I had been in Westport one week and I had already made a mom friend! I was so excited!

When I knew we were going to move into Westport, I went online on Facebook to look for mom groups to meet fellow moms. I was accepted to one. I went to one of the playdates at someone's house one Wednesday afternoon. I was shocked when I got there, because there were more than 15 moms with their toddlers and babies. I did not expect so many moms were not working! In Norwalk, the moms I met, most of them had gone back to work after their maternity leave had ended. At this playdate, all those moms were stay at home moms! Fantastic! All like me! This was going to be so much fun! I exchanged phones with the ones I got along with, in order to contact them to go on playdates once I moved in into the house in Westport. It was a bit strange that they all asked me where I lived. I explained to them in Norwalk and told them the offer on the house was accepted. They changed a bit their tone when I said Norwalk. Don't know why, but I didn't really pay attention to that as I was simply fascinated with so many moms that I could become friends with if they were like me, stay at home moms. I texted three of them to get together after I met them. Two never came back to me, and one I did see. We went on a playdate once. The next time I saw her, she ignored me and didn't even say hello. That was so strange. I had heard some rumors that moms in Westport could be quite snobby, but I didn't want to believe that. I know there are a lot of nice kind human beings in the world and prefer to believe in the kindness of people. That Facebook group never really posted many more playdates in winter so I never saw them again. The moms I met that didn't come back to me, I don't judge them. They may already have a lot of friends and don't have time for more. On the contrary, I had just moved in to town and was eager to meet other moms. Therefore I decided to create a new Facebook group called "Westport Stay at Home Moms of Babies and toddlers".

To create the group, I added my mom friends from Norwalk and Hannah, the only Westport mom I knew. Little by little, some other moms that saw the group online, requested to join and that's how I met Michelle and her husband Matt, who has also become one of my closest friends here. Her daughter Corrine and Nicole have become best friends. She was part of a different group for playdates as well, not in Facebook but Meetups. I went to several of the meetups that two other Westport moms created. Through that group I made as well new friends. That platform charged a fee to be part of it, so I invited the admins of that group, to join my Facebook group, and be admins of this group too, that was free. So they came to the along with the moms that were in that group, and the group became bigger. It also was more friendly user, as in Facebook groups we can post pictures, polls, reminders, etc. The group had reached approximately 40 members when they joined the group. I started to have more and more playdates every week. Meet more moms, and Nicole make more friends. Suddenly my agenda felt like the president's agenda! It was completely booked! I had a minimum of two playdates per day. I was having so much fun! All the moms I met were so nice. It was like moms Disneyland. Everyday having fun with friends. The best vacation ever. This was my new life? Really! Amazing. This completely started to change my mood and my mindset towards the topic of being a stay at home mom. This life is great! Sure, I miss work, but it is honestly starting to feel so far away now. So far behind in the past. Yes, the reason why I am not working is far from ideal, a brain tumor, but my new reality is not bad at all. The Facebook group started to grow exponentially as more and more moms joined and more and more moms started to do playdates created by them. Now we have playdates in houses, on the beach, in public places, etc. We also have now official events like moms night out, holidays we celebrate together and stroller walks if the weather allows. Not only are the moms making friends, but the husbands have gotten to meet each other and they are too now making dad friends. The group has become so big (160 members in 5 months) that I am now using the size of the group to get us some special discounts for our get togethers. I am so happy the Westport Stay At Home Moms group has opened the door for other moms and myself to make friends. Meaningful friends, from different backgrounds, different interests, different education, but with one thing in common which is be nice to each other and have fun with their toddlers.

Whilst the playdates are fun, the brain fatigue takes its toll. I put on a happy face with all my friends, but when I get home I let go and Simon often bears the brunt. Mood swings, extreme tiredness. It is very normal for me now to go to bed straight after dinner (or sometimes half way through).

There is one more side effect after my surgery I haven't mentioned before in the book. My brain sends the wrong signal to my bladder, telling it I need to empty my bladder, pee, when I don't really need to. So I go to the bathroom and basically not much comes out. I go once an hour. The first year after the surgery I wasn't paying any attention to this, as I had stronger side effects to worry about like the pain or learning how to read and write again. The drugs I had been taking gave me several different side effects including insomnia. One year after the surgery I started to notice how extremely often I was going to the bathroom day and night. It gave me insomnia because I would go to the bathroom once per hour at night. Imagine, falling asleep at 11, and then waking up at 12, 1, 2, 3, 4, 5, and so on to pee, and nothing comes out. It literally wakes me up. One of those times, I can't fall asleep again. There is the insomnia. I stay in bed from 1am to 5am trying to fall asleep. It had been months of me not sleeping well, but I was not working, so I could always recover a bad night of sleep next morning. I did tell my neurosurgeon, but about it and he said he had never heard of this side effect. It was clearly the reason though, as I did not have this problem before the surgery. He told me to see a urologist to see if there could be something done. I went, but I had just found out I was pregnant. The one drug that could maybe help, was not approved for pregnancy nor breastfeeding. So I would have to wait at least a year to even try it. During pregnancy my insomnia was not bothering me as I could continue to rest the next day. Once Nicole was born, it definitely was not bothering me at all, as with a newborn no one gets to sleep anyway. I would have to feed her so often, her feeding times were almost aligned with my bathroom schedule. Nicole is now 2 years old and she now sleeps through the night. Now she requires me awake and to have energy during the day. More than ever it is key for me to rest at night. The problem is, my brain continues to send the same wrong signal. So I'm suffering from insomnia at least 3-4 times a week. This is exhausting! I am constantly exhausted. I started the gym to see if being more tired at night would help me sleep through my wrong brain signals, but it didn't work. So a friend of mine recommended I try medical marihuana.

Medical Marihuana, really? I've never liked marijuana. I find it boring and it only makes me want to eat like a pig and sleep. Oh wait, sleep? The couple of times I tried it in France with friends I do remember it made me sleep like a baby. I stopped smoking cigarettes 8 years ago, which makes me hate smoking. So I couldn't smoke it. No way. Yuck! I told this to my friend and she recommended to go to a medical marihuana doctor and ask about different methods that exist, so I took an appointment.

The Medical Marihuana doctor was so nice and understanding. She told me she was so happy I found her, because it is exactly for cases like mine that she became licensed. A mother too, her baby girl was diagnosed with cancer years ago. Years of treatments, chemotherapies, different types of medicines, she tried it all, for more than a decade, and her little one didn't seem to be getting better. So she decided to get her Liscense and treat her daughter. She has had a life changing opportunity where her daughter can now go out and play with friends and attend school. If this mom had the strength to give medical Marihuana to an underage child and has made a positive change in her lifestyle, this could definitely help me too, right? After hearing my story and going through my medical records, she approved the license. I waited one month in order to get the paperwork to be able to go and buy the medical marihuana.

Once I had bought my first pills and tried it, the effect was amazing! Instead of going 6-7 times a night to the bathroom, I started to go only 3-4 times. That is a big change! 50% less. The first two weeks I only had insomnia one time. Only once! I was full of energy the next day. My brain fatigue levels the same, but my energy drastically better.

Simon was a bit more comfortable with this topic once I had met with the doctor and told him about her story and her child. I also insisted him to try once, because he had never smoked before he was thinking the side effect was so much stronger. Not sure, but I think he thought it was like mushrooms, or some stronger drug that makes you see things. Once he finally tried it he said:

"This is it?! What's all the fuss for? "

When he saw how mild it was, he was more ok with it. In addition, because its medical, you can control the amount you intake through pills instead of smoking. I can take very small dosages in order to help me to sleep, without making me tired or drowsy the next day, like sleeping pills. Two months after taking medical marihuana pills before sleeping, I rarely suffer from insomnia. The wrong signals to my brain seem to be significantly less with the pill. I only take it at night off course, so during the day I still use the bathroom every hour. I don't mind. I told my parents, neither of whom are fans of marihuana and to my surprise they were both very happy I had found a legal solution to my insomnia and both are completely on board with this. Who would of thought, I've always hated pot and now I'm officially licensed. Life is full of surprises!

Almost 8 months being settled in our new home, and I still have not received the money from Social Security. It's been months since the hearing and my approval, yet we have not been paid.

Surprisingly long. The money that we receive anyways will have to go directly to the private insurance and once that happens, they will start paying my benefits again. In the judge's ruling, I would have to appoint a legal representative to manage the check I would receive from Social Security due to my limitations with numbers and short term memory. My lawyer recommended Simon and he was approved for this role. That also means I can't talk to Social Security or ask any questions. Simon has to call, and I could help him as calling Social Security takes generally one hour wait time on the phone. Its not easy to wait so long with no news or update. Every time we call they don't have a concrete answer as to when we will receive the money that was approved. Still, I don't feel I have the right to complain because I'm receiving help.

My new happiness is not work. My new happiness is my little Nicole. I feel the Westport Stay At Home Moms have helped many moms make friends in town and give them happiness. The feeling that I have helped is what brings me joy now. The months I spent volunteering, creating platforms in Facebook that help other brain tumor patients and help moms make new mom friends. What all these platforms have in common is the fact of helping others. That is what is bringing me happiness. This is what I would like to continue to do. Help others.

I am a member of a different Facebook page in Westport called Westport Gift Economy, were neighbors share things they no longer want or need, and post them in the page, to see if anyone wants it. One of the admins of that page, Sonam, is also one of the admins in the WSAHM. I was so inspired by that concept, that I created a similar one, with a different name in Colombia. All this got me thinking, I would love to create a Non Profit to send toys and clothes to Colombia for children in need. That is going to be my next project. I know I have to maintain my energy though. I know I get brain fatigued and can't push myself too much. I definitely will give this idea a try. I want to bring joy to people. My new purpose in life is to help others, bringing them together, at my own pace, part time. I would like to help people smile.

I know it might sound like I am very socially active and doing many different things daily, but that is not really the case. I still get brain fatigue and will continue to get it the rest of my life. Sleeping well every night has helped a lot, but still, I do control my energy levels. I moderate my calendar of activities to always have resting days in the middle. In addition, every weekend Simon supports me by taking care of Nicole and I use the weekend to recover. Therefore we don't do much on the weekends. During the week as well, by the time Simon arrives home, I am exhausted. He is such a great husband and father. From time to time, not too often, I do still get a little sad. When I have some time for myself, I still cry alone in the car, remembering my past, what I lost and the person I used to be. I guess it's normal to still get sad sometimes. I still remember the feeling of walking down the corridors of Jackson Memorial reading "8" every number, and the "crack crack" of my brain and the coloring for hours sitting on my sofa in the house in Coral Gables. Memories that will always be with me, with Simon, and my family and friends that lived that time with me.

I am so happy now. I like the new me. It has taken years to get to know the new me. A me that is officially disabled, partially dumb and partially blind. I have come to accept the new me and I like myself again. Yes, I have changed, but I have gained so much more too. I am more patient, humble, open to other people's differences. I don't judge before trying to understand the person. How could I understand how much there is to someone's life before we get to know them. I mean, look at me. There is so much that I have lived in my short life. I love being a mom. I never imagined how much happiness it would give me. I don't miss my past life anymore. I am no longer nostalgic of what I lost. I now see how much I have gained. I am looking forward to my new reality. Patiently, one project at a time, one friend at a time and helping one person at a time. I want to dedicate my life to helping others. I also want to dedicate my life to my little Nicole and Simon. I am so grateful of the support I have received from so many people, that love me or simply just know me. It is time to pay back, and support others. I feel I have rediscovered life after a brain tumor, a new life and I love it!

CHAPTER NINE

TWO PRINCESSES – BY SIMON

Two princesses…I'll come back to that part. Nathalie has been asking me to write this chapter for some time now and it's not because I didn't want to that I failed to pick up the pen and write. I never knew how to start. I had a name and that was it. I mean, how honest would she want me to be? Who am I really writing this for? It started as something for our soon-to-be-born daughter, Nicole, so that she could look back and one day understand something of what her mother had to go through. But now it feels like the story perhaps has a greater purpose, to share what it might mean to others who are facing a similar journey or perhaps are just interested.

So I will start. When I walked into the recovery room with Philippe (Nathalie's father), my heart sank. To see her lying there, her head covered in a big bandage, with a huge splint on her right forearm and various cables connected to various monitors, I felt helpless. A husband's role is to protect his wife, and there I was, watching in a blur.

You see, the day Nathalie called me to say they had found something and we needed to go to the ER right away, I wasn't sure what to think. I guess I wasn't thinking too much at that point. I'm not going to repeat what Nathalie has written about that part, only to say that the day we met Dr. Smith it was a surreal experience. We walked into that room with our health, a nice lifestyle in Miami and two very good salaries. The experience was short, but not so sweet. I just held her hand. I didn't know what else to do. "Will there be any side effects?" I asked.

"There's a twenty percent probability of temporary loss of peripheral eyesight; only a two percent chance it will be permanent," he said.

So I thought, *It sounds pretty straightforward then. She will be fine.*

As we left the room, we passed a lady sitting in the waiting room. She had a large sutured cut on her left frontal lobe. Her head was partly shaven, and it was clear that she had recently undergone some kind of surgery. I didn't put two and two together. I didn't for one second think that was what Naths was about to go through. I was imagining a keyhole surgery. Actually, I don't know what I was imagining. My mind was blank. The relaxed attitude of the doctor didn't give me any cause for alarm and the preparation was focused on hospital pajamas and a new pair of Crocs, instead of making a note of banking passwords or if we had sufficient insurance.

With the in-laws in town, I felt a bit more support. They are always very supportive. But it still hadn't hit me. When I told my boss at work, I think she was more shocked than I was. In fact, everyone at work was great with me, always asking how Nathalie was.

So when I saw Nathalie lying there, in that bed, not really able to speak, with a big egg on her head, it was like I had just run into a wall. She didn't remember my name at first. She recognized her father immediately, but I was a bit of a blur. We had to rotate spaces, so Antonella came in, and I went out, and then Philippe…this went on for several hours until it was 9:30 at night. I told them to go home to rest. I would stay until she moved up to ICU. We had been waiting for a bed for over five hours. She was sleeping most of the time due to the morphine, and I was constantly telling the nurses about her low pain threshold.

We finally moved up to ICU and I said I was going to leave so that she could rest and I would come back when visiting hours resumed. At that point, something happened. It was as if there was nothing wrong with her, and she stared straight through me and called me "fucking selfish" and then slipped back into the same drowsy state. I didn't know what to feel. Normally I would have resented the attack and it would have been the trigger for an argument, but I didn't. My thinking was, *What use would I be if I was here, tired as well? How could I stay strong for her?* I guess I was being selfish. So I asked for a blanket and slumped into a reclining chair by the side of her bed.

Every thirty minutes or so, she cried out, and I jumped up and held her hand and asked a nurse to administer more morphine. This went on throughout the night until I was kicked out. There was a gap in visiting hours when the doctors made rounds in the ICU. This was at about six in the morning. I drove myself home to get showered and came back again. I just wasn't expecting all of this.

I stayed at her side for the rest of her hospital stay. I couldn't leave her. She was so helpless, lying there. I felt drained, emotionally drained. I wasn't there for the first story of the eights, as I had gone home to shower and change as I did each morning. When I saw her write for the first time or try to say her birthday, the shock became a cold reality that I had not been expecting. Was this how she would be for the rest of our lives? What went wrong? This was more than a 20 percent probability of peripheral vision loss.

"She is suffering from Gerstmann syndrome," the doctor said.

This meant nothing to me, so I Googled it. "It will get better; it is normal." If it is so fucking normal, why didn't I know about it before? We all wanted to make her feel comfortable and took turns sitting next to her in the grandiose hospital room.

Nathalie pointed at the blinds, which were vertical slats covering a blurred glass pane. Not articulating what she wanted to say, she continued to point, so I opened them. "No," she said and continued to point at them with more frustration. So I started to feel frustrated for not understanding. I closed them again. "No," she said again, still pointing. "Pillow," she said. She had wanted me to adjust her pillow. Then I felt a pain inside. It was difficult to see and hear the girl I love so much unable to do or ask for what she wanted.

It was an emotional week. I cried many times. I felt helpless. I couldn't keep her safe; I couldn't make it better. The moment they took off the bandage, I was shocked. A twelve-inch cut on her head, like something out of a movie. Like the lady in the reception, but in a different location. *Will this ever heal?* I asked myself.

The day of the operation, I was like a switchboard, calling Nathalie's mom, my mom, and my dad, and sitting with Philippe and Antonella while we waited. When the doctor came in and said everything went well, she was fine and was now in recovery, I had no expectation of what was to come; I mean, I have had two surgeries on my left knee, both with general anesthetic, and I was fine.

We all cried when we heard the news. We would get to see

her in thirty minutes. The surgery had been quick, two hours. It was due to last four. When she finally focused and recognized me, I said, "Hello, Princess."

She responded, "Hello, Princess."

"Do you know my name?"

She looked confused and replied, "Princess." Had she forgotten? She closed her eyes again. She also thought we were in the year 1800 something, so I didn't worry too much. I just thought it was cute. This continued for a couple of days, where my nickname had changed from Monkey to Princess.

As you may have read already, we were in the process of putting a pool in. When I got back from the hospital, I found that they had snapped all the branches on the trees to get access to install a new fence. I got mad, with a mixture of tiredness, emotion and anger at the ignorant workmanship. The foreman had been supportive once I told him about Nathalie. He changed scheduling as much as he could and always asked how she was. He even texted me last month, over a year later, to ask how she was. Very nice.

Anyway, I needed to get the new air conditioning installed before Naths would come home. We got that sorted, but I was juggling that and the hospital, and I found it hard emotionally.

Naths was demanding, as she was vulnerable. Friends were all messaging or calling me, and I was trying my best to keep family updated. Never underestimate the support network around you.

It's 1 in the morning as I'm writing this, fifteen months from the surgery. As I look back, I still feel the raw emotion from that day, week, first four months. I never expected I would experience something like that in my life and I would not wish it on anyone.

My poor baby has been through so much with all of this and I still feel as helpless as I did that day.

A week after the surgery, Nathalie was back home. We had to make adjustments to make her more comfortable. She got flowers and magazines, which were a lovely thought, but she couldn't read them. She couldn't watch TV; she couldn't add two plus two. She was finding this all funny. I laughed, but I didn't know what to feel. I was scared.

She went to the kitchen to make a cup of tea. She grasped the kettle in her right hand and lifted it. "I know I need to do something, but I don't know what." Her cognitive functioning was not there. At this point, we banned her from the kitchen altogether. It was too dangerous for her.

We were still oblivious of things to come. In 2015, we spent $18,000 on medical bills. We couldn't afford to live in our beautiful house any more. We had to make some changes. Nathalie had always been the main breadwinner and I was kind of OK with that. There were times my male ego kicked in, but, generally, I didn't mind. She had worked hard to get where she was and came through some tough moments, and she deserved it.

In our first week home, I realized that I needed to pay the credit cards. I didn't have the passwords and she couldn't remember them. Naths had taken care of all of this before. Fuck! After some trial and error, we managed and I paid them, with a small late fee, which I didn't tell her.

The best thing about this whole thing was that Nathalie said yes to everything. She was calm, enjoying the simple things in life in between being in pain. I, for once, was making the decisions. I was the man of the house and my wife was happy with all of them! This didn't last for long. As the months progressed, her emotions changed. As she became more aware, the drugs wore off, the frustrations kicked in, and she was cognizant of not being able to add or remember. She got stuck when she spoke, suffered from insomnia and was insecure around other people. She could still speak three languages, but she couldn't articulate a clear sentence in any language. She got angry quickly.

To the outside world, I was coping admirably. I was amazing. On the inside, I was breaking down. My tiredness kicked in and I snapped back, forgetting what she had been through or not understanding how she must be coping. I didn't talk about it and I didn't know what to do. Some friends were better than others. Perhaps they didn't know what to say or do. Some disappeared. I was disappointed and I was sad for her. Sharing your situation with your close friends before and along the way and setting up their expectations is an important piece of advice I would give, as you will need them on both sides. This includes family. Family will say they understand, but they won't.

Some reactions shocked me, but I didn't say anything. The mood swings continued. Sometimes there were more than others. I could escape to the office at this point, but I couldn't really, as I was faced with many daily question. I had to smile and give the politically correct answer to people who I knew really didn't give a shit, but they felt that they had to ask. Others were genuine and I was more open with them.

I didn't know what to do to help Naths. I didn't know how to help her pain. The emotions were running high and low. She was crying, shouting, crying. She was trapped inside and this thing didn't seem to be improving.

The first visit was at three weeks, then four weeks, then one month, then six months, then one year, then 18 months. We are now at 15 months and she is not how she was before. In fact, it is highly likely that she will ever be as she was before. We are less than two months away from our first child, Nicole, and the pregnancy has added to her ongoing fatigue. This roller coaster of emotions has been exacerbated by our move to Connecticut and I feel that I isolated her. She is trapped in her mind and now trapped in the countryside. At least in Miami, she had friends.

We moved because of me. My job. The timing wasn't great. In fact, it was shit. I agonized over the decision. She said yes straightaway, but I was twenty-four hours behind her. I wish we had stayed, for her. I don't think I was strong enough. I don't think I was selfish. We made the decision together, but perhaps I didn't really consider the consequences. I thought she was on the brink of full recovery, that therapy would continue and she would get a job again. I don't know if we had stayed if her brain would have recovered more.

We were past the six-month learning curve peak (some say six months; some say one year), but I look in her eyes now and I see pain, sadness, and loneliness, a void that I could fill in the hospital, and now I cannot. Her passion in life was working, and it was taken from her. Now that she's pregnant, life will take a different course once more, but the consequence of that one thirty-minute meeting with the doctor changed the course of our lives together forever.

I have so many questions. Did he make a mistake? Was this always the plan? If she hadn't gone skiing and fallen, how would we have discovered this? Would things have been worse? What if we had stayed in Miami? I kind of feel helpless again. The fatigue will get you. The insurance doesn't understand that or want to understand that. It creates frustrations. Our arguments are not rational. The memory loss is apparent and there is no outlet.

Each day I see my two princesses, one waiting to be born to a world that she will make her own, and the other whom I adore so much, looking half of what she used to be emotionally. Do I love her any less? *No.* I love her more. I have more admiration for her than ever before. I am so proud of what she has come through and how she continues to be positive and moves forward. Ever since I met her almost five years ago, I have looked up to her, learned from her and adored her. She still teaches me things each day and I feel helpless in return, unable to protect and make things better as a husband should.

I am a believer that if you work hard enough, you can achieve anything. The brain is a muscle. It needs to be worked. Therapy is important; release is important; support is important. My favorite song of all time is "Don't Give Up" by Philippe Gabriel. I never knew how relevant that song would be to this situation.

The thing about emotion is that it envelops you. Like a wave washing over you, it controls you. They say that patience is a virtue, but it is easy to forget patience when everything looks fine on the outside. The brain tumor's side effects that Nathalie suffered are all on the inside, but looking at her, you wouldn't think anything was wrong. There is no visible scar. Her hair has grown back; her face is normal. So appearances can be deceiving and being around her daily, I can easily forget what she has been through and what she was suffering inside.

This malpractice from my side could easily be avoided by just reminding myself each day that I need to be patient. Perhaps her response to things is due to the cognitive deficit, the short-term memory loss or the fatigue. Each time, I should remove myself from the situation and take the defensive emotion out and I need to consider my response or my explanation, as Nathalie is perhaps not as controlled as she would want.

It's difficult because I forget, not because I want to forget or because I don't care, but because life takes over, this perception that

I mentioned tricks my mind perhaps. Even the fact that I am automatically writing this in the second person probably tells me something, that I need to be more accountable…learning how to communicate again is the key.

Communication is at the heart of any relationship. Yes, love is important, but love can generate both emotional fears and pleasures. Communication conquers all and when you are suffering from side effects that inhibit your ability to effectively communicate, then the other partner needs to step up, and this is where I feel I have failed. I have always been a passive person, trying to avoid conflict where possible; however, what I learned about myself through this is that I have to learn how to communicate better and now I manage conflict much better.

The hardest thing for Nathalie to accept through all this is that none of it was her fault. Neither of us believes in any god; we believe in science. We don't know how the tumor occurred. We don't know why the side effects she suffered scored eight out of ten in strength. We don't know why her eyesight or her full cognitive abilities haven't come back.

Nathalie now considers herself dumb. an opinion that I profusely disagree with. She has always been someone I look up to and adore, someone that I learn from, who has a high capability for reasoning, and she hasn't lost this part, and I have not lost this admiration. My role in this is to keep the fire burning. A fire needs fuel to be strong, and I have to put the logs on, keep giving encouragement, keep giving praise for the efforts to improve. I have to be patient, detach myself emotionally so I can be there for her, and stay strong. I adapt our surroundings so she is safe and doesn't need to be constantly reminded of the areas she struggles with. For example, when we walk where there are people, I always walk on the right side. Even though she won't see me there, I know it keeps her safer so that she won't bump into some stranger. But patience is something I need to work on more.

For any partners or family members who are about to support an operation, here are eight things that I learned that you should consider:

Patience—take a breath. Remember that your loved one might not be able to articulate what he or she really wants to say (the blinds examples). The outside might look "normal," so how you interpret the message needs to be through patience and asking questions.

Listen—don't pass judgment. Listen when he or she is ready to speak. Just be there. There will be complaints from noises in the head, lighting too bright, voices too loud. Just go with it.

Speak—share your feelings with someone. Don't bottle them up. It will impact you emotionally, and bottled-up emotion can release, much like shaking a soda bottle before opening it.

Learn—learn about your loved one's new habits—all the hobbies that we enjoyed together stopped temporarily, and some have completely gone. Naths started enjoying coloring.

Plan—financially this will probably impact you more that you think. Job loss, insurance, copays, therapies—these might not stop at three weeks, six weeks, one month, one year, eighteen months. The little things that we take for granted, such as passwords, thinking practically, planning together. Don't leave any big decisions, as your loved one will likely contribute to them without really knowing what he or she is committing to.

Laugh—enjoy the ride, release, and laugh. Laughter releases endorphins, which create the feeling of happiness. Moments that can make you break down and cry can be turned into laughter. The night before the operation, I slept at Nathalie's side in the hospital, subjected to the telenovela coming from the lady's TV in the cubicle next door and the worst McDonald's food that I had ever eaten. Nathalie, Philippe, Antonella, and I were sitting there when the doctor came in and stuck Polos on her face. With this was the stark realization that she was about to have brain surgery, but we laughed because she had Polos (Life Savers in the USA) stuck on her face.

Love—this one sounds obvious, but just being there, holding a hand, changing your agenda to give support and show compassion, can be a big emotional support—more than you think. You don't want your loved one worrying about your agenda. Cancel everything in the first month if you can.

Ask—the doctors won't volunteer the information to you. The nurses are somewhat better. Ask, and document everything, not only from a diligence point of view but for the insurance company. You will need to fight for Social Security benefits or long-term disability and pay medical bills, which will likely be wrong at some point. Keep a ledger and record everything; it will save headaches when you are trying to manage everything else.

So going back to that night before the operation, lying there next to my wife in the hospital bed, with the Polos stuck to her head, it dawned on me that this thing was a very big deal, I mean, it was brain surgery. I don't think either of us really slept that night. We were awoken at one in the morning for a detailed MRI to prep for the surgery, and then again at five to be washed, before being taken down to prep at six thirty, which is when they finally listened to me about her name being spelled incorrectly. Make sure you check all the details on your partner's records, as the slightest mistake will cause you problems in the long term. Don't take this for granted. All humans make errors, brain tumor or not.

Would we have slept better had we been better prepared?

Probably not. Just being there helped the process. Mindfulness is a topic you may or may not have heard of. It's an interesting subject about being present. Do you listen, or are you hearing? You are the support network now. You need to be there. Everything else in life becomes secondary.

My employer was supportive of me. While giving me paid leave as a caregiver was not an option unless I took my holidays, I was allowed to work from home for as long as I needed to. This did help, but I didn't always find myself present. As they say in Brazil, I had one eye on the cat and one eye on the fish. If you try to do both, you will fail at both. Just be present.

I have always been a good planner, I think. I found it easy to set an agenda for the six different pills that Naths needed to take across various intervals throughout the day, including at two, four, and six in the morning in the early days. Antonella was great and took turns with me in the first week so I could sleep during the early morning ones sometimes. We had been prepared with one thing, the shower seat. "You won't need that," I said, not wanting to pay the twenty dollars or whatever it cost…I'm glad we did buy it though.

I said in the beginning that I would come back to the two princesses part…

As we start our next big planning expedition, our greatest roles in life are yet to come. In four weeks' time, our first child will be born. We are expecting a little girl and she will become my second princess. It is my hope that I keep my two princesses safe to the best of my ability. That means supporting, teaching, loving and listening to them. I hope that my daughter never has to go through the trauma that Naths has been through, but she can read back through this book and learn and understand how important it is to be kind and companionate, to always be honest, to treat others as she would like to be treated, and to have patience and to never presume or take people for granted.

The day that Nathalie told me she was pregnant, I felt so proud. I was so happy that I cried. I was so proud of her after everything that she had gone through. This was a new beginning for her and for us, the next chapter in our lives. But, another little princess in my life…how the hell would I cope with that?

Life is all about learning, and this is something we will be learning together. So as throughout the surgery I needed to be there to learn my role and my place, to be a support and help Nathalie read and write and do math, I will be called on once more. This time, I can't wait!

I have learned a lot about myself in this past year. I've had many reflections on my past and things I have done more so than the things I haven't. I had thought I was patient, but I hadn't really been tested. Trauma tests you; loss tests you, and while we will all experience bumps in the road—losing a job, losing a girlfriend, or quarreling with a friend—it is how we learn from these situations and become stronger that is important. What I have learned is that without patience, it is much harder to learn.

For whatever value my words might add to your situation or to help prepare you, remember this: each situation is its own. Ours was certainly not textbook—fewer than 2% of all brain tumors, so not much is known. Is this a cheap excuse for not being prepared or being informed? Probably, but, in the end, the important things for us were patience and love.

CHAPTER TEN

LESSONS AND ADVICE

We all have lessons in life. We learn from our own experiences, from others' experiences and from things we do correctly as well as our mistakes; tough moments, happy moments and tragic ones too. The saying "prepare for the worst; expect the best" could not be more true. Even if we know this, we definitely don't make significant changes in our lives unless we have to. I would like to share with you some advice for not only if you or a loved one has been diagnosed with a brain tumor, but for life in general. I hope my lessons, my mistakes, and my good decisions can help you in your life.

Be grateful and thankful and don't expect anything from others. I've learned that the moment we start expecting gestures or things from others, we open the possibility of being disappointed. When someone, family or not, offers help and support, economical or emotional, when you don't expect it, you will always feel grateful.

If you actually feel you deserve or expect those types of gestures from others, you stop being grateful and can actually start to feel disappointed when you don't receive them.

I felt thankful for the people I expected support from, like my family. But people I was not expecting anything, surprised me with small gestures that filled my life with joy. For example, I was Nani's boss when I worked at Diageo and we continued to be friends. Since the surgery, she has been one my greatest supports, and during the recovery, she was absolutely incredible to me. Who would have thought that she would be taking care of me when I couldn't be left alone in the house? Tasos, our Greek friend, was unconditionally supportive throughout my recovery too. He visited often and stocked me with gummy bears. He always made me laugh because he made fun of my lack of math skills, which I also found hilarious at the time. I received flowers from unexpected people, like Alberto Gavazzi (the President for Latin America in Diageo). I was so pleasantly surprised that we called them the great Gavazzi's flowers.

While I felt so grateful, I also felt hurt or disappointed with people who didn't do much. Again, it all came down to me expecting certain gestures from certain people, and, therefore, I felt disappointed. I didn't feel angry or anything negative toward them, but definitely didn't feel grateful.

If you can choose between these two types of feelings, grateful versus disappointed, grateful will give you more happiness in life. You can't control other people's intentions, but you can choose to control how you feel about them. So don't expect anything, and you will be grateful for anything you receive.

Laugh twice as much as you cry.
I think that not knowing that I had the possibility of having such strong, lifelong side effects allowed me to laugh and enjoy every single moment post-surgery. I was lucky that I didn't realize this would be for life, so I took it lightly and enjoyed every single moment of it, from not knowing how to write my name to listening to the birds in the street. Thinking back, it's quite amazing that those

first six months were super fun and filled with new life experiences, and I enjoyed them all. I laughed at them all. I did cry, but when I look back, it was a happy time.

If you can choose between making it a happy time in your life or a depressing one, why not try to enjoy it? Why not convert the bad into good? I'm not saying it's easy, but we will face so many tragedies, deaths, so traumas, losses, and difficult moments, why not try to laugh and enjoy some of them. We can at least can try.

Reinvent yourself.
Plan your life path, but know that life will have a plan of its own for you. Happiness, fulfilment, and accomplishment will be a mix of achieving what you planned, worked for, and desired and surpassing the obstacles you didn't plan for, ask for, or deserve.

Having the mental flexibility to reinvent yourself, your goals, and what brings you joy and meaning in life will be the strength you need to continue building your life path, without breaking you when things get in the way. Don't just hope for a better moment, create it, work for it, and make it happen. Life doesn't happen for you; you make it happen.

Don't make "Everything will be fine," "It could have been worse," "I understand you" comments.
Just listen and support others. Keep the light fortune-cookie messages to yourself. No, you do not understand the other person, as you are not going through this. Even if everything will be fine, it's not what the person wants to hear. No, you don't understand. How could you?

When people feel helpless and sad about what they are living, they only want to be heard, listened to and hugged. Don't solve the problem for them. Don't give them a long list of rational solutions that they don't want to listen to. Just look at them, hug them, let them cry if they need to. That is more support and will make them feel more comforted than any list of solutions.

Don't try to put yourself in other people's shoes as you cannot feel what they feel, not even if you are going through the exact same things. Lives are too different, as are pasts and presents, and you will never ever be able to feel exactly the same thing another feels.

Learn to forgive.
Everyone makes mistakes, and so will you. Life is long even though we feel its short. You will have enough time to make people happy, make people cry, do the right thing and also make mistakes, and so will the people around you. I doubt there are many people in the world who want to hurt you on purpose in a rationally planned way. The closer you are to others, meaning family or very close friends, the greater the chance they will hurt you. Guaranteed this will happen.

When it does, stop and think about whether they hurt you on purpose. Did they say or do what they did to purposely hurt you, or was it the consequence of a decision they made? Maybe it was the wrong decision, but it probably wasn't intentionally planned and thought of to hurt you. So forgive when someone hurts you. This is the only way you can be happy.

In my family, there are members who have not forgiven and I don't see what good can come from that. It may take a bit of time, but forgive. If I hadn't forgiven and reunited with relatives, I would have lived a life without a mother or father and Antonella, people who now bring me immense love, support and happiness. Don't miss out on life and the great opportunities of happy moments with your loved ones because you are unable to move on and forgive. At some point, you will also be in a position of making a mistake and needing to be forgiven.

Only you can decide if you want to create a happy life for yourself. Take it in your hands to make yourself and others happy by letting go of mistakes. Use the opportunity to learn and don't repeat the same ones again. Learn and move one. Learn and forgive.

Consciously enjoy the good moments in life.
Don't take the good moments for granted. Unfortunately, sooner or later, we will all get sick, a loved one will die, and you will have bad

economic times. Sooner or later—that is the big question and only life will tell you when those moments will come. So consciously enjoy the good ones! There will be more good ones than bad, but sometimes life piles them up together or spreads them out. Who knows?

Just remember to enjoy them and feel thankful they are there. I'm not saying to panic that bad things will happen, but to consciously enjoy the good things. For example, I had always had great health and I took that for granted. I never felt grateful at all. My health has now significantly impacted my life, and only now do I realize how important it was. So as a lesson, even with a hole in my head now, I consciously make sure I remember how lucky I am because I am healthy with my hole in my head.

Enjoy the money and enjoy the lack of it.
Enjoy luxuries when you can afford them—travel, hotels, restaurants, clothes and anything else you define as luxury. But be as happy with them as you are without them. Be flexible in knowing that material things give you a short-term hype, but, believe me, if you are happy with them, then you can be without them. Learning how to enjoy the free things as much as the paid ones is the key to balance. We have become a far-too materialistic society.

Save.
Every dollar you have in a savings is worth at least triple its value in peace of mind. We live in a society of material goods, technological innovations we feel the need to have, places around the world we want to travel to, and excessive amounts of clothes to choose from. We tend to save a bit, but we don't really plan for the worst. With savings, I was fortunate I didn't have to worry about the thousands of dollars we paid for surgery, therapies, and drugs. The peace of mind from being able to pay for the short-term needs was invaluable. Now that I am unable to work, I do wish I would have saved even more.

Get life insurance while you are healthy and young.
We think we are invincible and will stay healthy forever, until we are not, until it is too late. We tend think about life insurance when we have children, not before. With our generation waiting to have children at an older age than our previous generation, we are at a higher risk of having something in our health records. My premium to buy it now is through the roof! If only I had bought life insurance before the brain tumor.

The following are craniotomy-related lessons and advice:

Don't expect your family and friends to understand what you are going through.
Prepare to explain as much as you feel you need or want to. I found out that most of the people I was surrounded by, including my closest friends and family members, did not research my brain tumor or its side effects, causes, or treatments. When you do the research, because you will probably become a hard-core researcher driven by your curiosity, this doesn't mean that others will. Once you have read all the books and papers and web pages on the topic and have become an expert, remember that the circle of people in your life won't know anything about it. Don't presume they understand or know anything.

I've noticed that when I have conversations with others, thinking that they understand my side effects, they sometimes don't even believe they are real. Take it as your job to try to explain to them. As they probably won't understand even with detailed explanations, send them links and videos. Hopefully they will read some, but even when you send them information, it doesn't mean they will read it.

Every individual will react differently to what you are living. They won't go through what you are going through and you can't expect them to guess or understand if you don't explain. When you feel others don't understand you, it can make you feel more isolated and alone. Avoid this feeling by teaching the people you want to teach what you are living. The sooner you do this, the sooner you set others on the journey with you, and the more they will support and understand you. In my case, I shared it with very few people and now I feel that people don't understand me, but I feel like it's too late to let them know.

Ask, ask, ask.
Doctors gave me very little information. Ask questions, and research prior to making any decisions and definitely get a second opinion. Even if it will lead you to make the same decision, you can be sure it's the correct one with more facts.

Plan items prior going into surgery.
1. Have a plan A and a plan B of people to take care of you in your home after surgery, if needed. I was lucky that I was married, my family was there and Simon was allowed to work from home for a month after my surgery. If I had been single or he couldn't have been home, I could not have taken care of myself, cooked, or even be by myself for the first two months.
2. Write down on a piece of paper, and I mean *paper*, all your passwords, e-mail accounts, bank accounts, and bills you have to pay.

    After my surgery, Simon had to help me recover every password of every single item online, as I couldn't remember any of them. I was the one who managed our bank account and bills, and we had to redo everything as I didn't remember any of them. If I had been single, I wouldn't have been able to pay for water or electricity on my own. Share the information with someone you trust. Hopefully you won't need it, but if you do, it is very practical to have it!
3. Preparation is difficult because the side effects are different from person to person and from tumor to tumor. I hadn't discovered that there were online communities on Facebook

for meningiomas, which have been great. I wish I had known prior to surgery.

4. Get a plastic shower stool.

5. Depending on the location of your scar, pillows will be a complicated item to find in order for you to sleep well. I bought a triangular one that kept me more upright than a normal pillow, which helped me to sleep.

6. Baby shampoo. You won't be allowed to shower your hair in the hospital, but a couple of days after you get back home, you will.

7. Health insurance. Make sure you ask your health insurance what is covered and keep the copies of every bill. One year after the surgery, I keep getting bills with mistakes that they needed to correct. It seemed like a never-ending task. Try to get the information of not only the hospital and your surgeon to be covered by your insurance, but also nurses, anesthesiologist, MRIs, and so on. Even if the hospital is covered, some stuff may not be, and you can get high bills that you have to pay 100%.

8. Check your disability insurance! What does it cover, and for how long? For example, do you know the difference between "any occupation" and "own occupation"? Get the details in writing.

Hospital list:

1. Warm Crocs! They are easy to put on and take off. This was, by far, the best item I took to the hospital. Hospitals are cold and so is the floor. The thick plastic insulates without the need for socks, and they are easy to wash and clean.

2. For women, nightgowns so that you don't have to take shorts or pants on and off when you go to the bathroom. In addition, look for short-sleeve ones, so the sleeve doesn't bother the IV that you will have on your arm.

3. Chapstick, cream, and phone charger.

4. Sunglasses, as you may be sensitive to light after surgery.

WHAT'S NEXT?

I know now that life can get sweeter and better after a brain tumor. I know now, that life can still bring you happiness no matter what you lose. Challenges, extremely difficult ones will come our way at one point or the other. We will lose some of the people we love, we will lose physical abilities, age will start affecting us and no matter how prepared we think we are, we will never be prepared enough to confront loss. We will fall but we must stand up again, because it is so worth it. Is it so worth standing back up again because life will bring happy moments again. The love we receive in life is greater, stronger, and more often than the sad moments. The level of profound love I feel for my little Nicole, my husband and my family and friends is what gives me the strength to smile every day. Happiness comes and goes, sadness comes and goes, but love, true love is always there.

CHAPTER ELEVEN

PICTURES

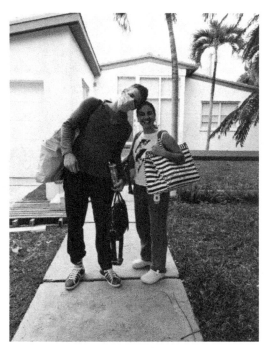

LEAVING TO THE HOSPITAL.

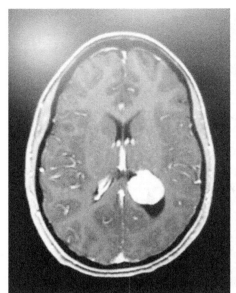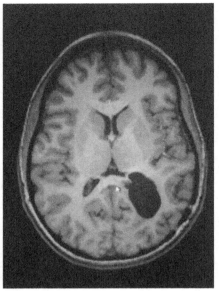

NATHALIE'S MRI 2015, BEFORE AND AFTER CRANIOTOMY

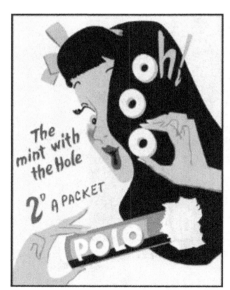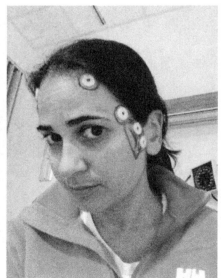

POLO JOKE FROM SIMON

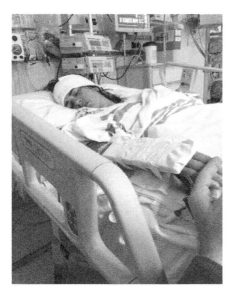

ICU AFTER SURGERY

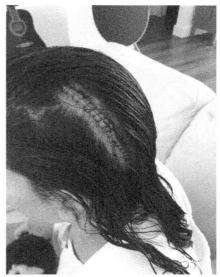

SCAR AFTER SURGERY

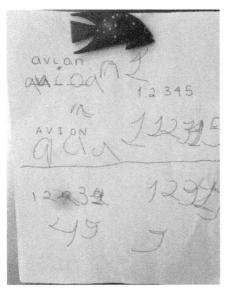

HANDWRITING AFTER SURGERY

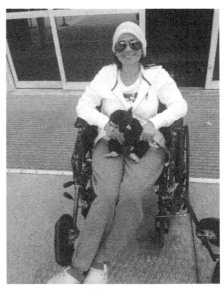

LEAVING THE HOSPITAL